Foreword

The decision of Harvey Cushing to leave general surgery and concentrate on the infant field of central nervous system surgery was in retrospect a landmark in the history of neurosurgery. His concentrated work, and also that of his colleague Walter Dandy, originated with the desires of both pioneers to understand surgical anatomy and neurophysiology. The fundamental knowledge and surgical techniques that they provided became the standard of excellence for several generations of neurosurgeons; so much so that the general belief was that the surgical techniques could not be improved upon.

Twenty-five to thirty years ago microtechniques began to appear in a few surgical research centers, they were then gradually applied to clinical neurosurgery and have contributed to a new level of understanding in surgical anatomy and neurophysiology. We are now fortunate to have a new standard of morbidity and mortality in the surgical treatment of intrathecal aneurysms, angiomas, and tumors. It has been said that microneurosurgery was reaching its limits, especially when treating lesions in and around the cavernous sinus and skull base; those lesions notorious for involvement of the dural and extradural compartments, with a tendency to infiltrate adjacent nerves and blood vessels. The dangers of uncontrollable hemorrhage from the basal sinuses and post-operative CSF rhinorrhea appeared unsurmountable. The lateral aspects of the petro-clival region have been of interest to a few pioneering ENT surgeons and neurosurgeons but the cavernous sinus in most respects has remained the final unconquered summit.

There have been some admirable approaches and results in surgery of the cavernous sinus, but broad clinical experience and precise surgical anatomic descriptions were missing; Professor Dolenc now presents such a pioneering work on the microanatomy and surgical compartments of this complex region. In addition, he provides new insight into the hemodynamic control of the petrous and intracavernous segments of the carotid artery, hemostatic control of the venous sinuses, and techniques for avoiding CSF rhinorrhea. The clinical sections convincingly demonstrate the effectiveness of this approach and characterize some of the remaining unsolved problems. There is no doubt that this type of microsurgical anatomy study is a new step in the 100 year history of neurosurgery. Finally, this work reconfirms the necessity for future generations of neurosurgeons to work in the microsurgery laboratory; not only for understanding the surgical anatomy, but to acquire the considerable technical skills necessary to perform surgical approaches of this complexity.

Zürich, August 10, 1989   *M. G. Yaşargil*

Vinko V. Dolenc

Anatomy and Surgery of the Cavernous Sinus

Foreword by Mahmut G. Yaşargil

Springer-Verlag Wien New York

Vinko V. Dolenc, M.D., Ph.D.
Professor and Chairman
University Department of Neurosurgery
University Medical Center
Ljubljana, Slovenia, Yugoslavia

Printed in Yugoslavia by Tiskarna Ljudske Pravice, YU-61000 Ljubljana

The use of registered names, trademarks, etc. in the publication does not imply, even in the absence of a specific statement, that such names are exempt from the relevant protective laws and regulations and therefore free for general use.

Product Liability: The publisher can give no guarantee for information about drug dosage and application thereof contained in this book. In every individual case the respective user must check its accuracy by consulting pharmaceutical literature.

With 182 Figures (126 in color)

ISBN 3-211-82155-4 Springer-Verlag Wien-New York
ISBN 0-387-82155-4 Springer-Verlag New York-Wien

Acknowledgments

I should like to extend my thanks to Ms Jasna Ostanek for all the time and care that she devoted to the editorial work throughout the preparation of the text. I am grateful to Thomas Wascher, M.D., for his valuable contribution to the initial text. Special thanks are due to Mr Bojan P. Moll, to John Kagi, M.D., and to Dianne Jones, M.D., for reading the text.

I am particulary grateful to Ms Jolanda Kofol, professional medical photographer, and to Mr Bogo Zrimšek, professional medical illustrator, for preparing the figures.

The indispensable help of medical student David Čokl and Borut Prestor, M.D., in the preparation of fresh cadaver specimens for microanatomical dissections, is gratefully acknowledged.

Vinko V. Dolenc

Contents

Abbreviations

Cranial nerves

ON	Optic nerve
III	Oculomotor nerve
IV	Trochlear nerve
V	Trigeminal nerve
GG	Gasserian ganglion
V1	Ophthalmic division
V2	Maxillary division
V3	Mandibular division
Vm	Motor branch of the trigeminal nerve
VI	Abducens nerve

Internal carotid artery

ICA	Internal carotid artery
(AL)	Anterior loop
(ML)	Medial loop
(LL)	Lateral loop
(PL)	Posterior loop

Other structures

A	Aneurysm
ACA	Anterior cerebral artery
ACoA	Anterior communicating artery
ACP	Anterior clinoid process
ACT	Anterior clinoid tip
AICS	Anterior intercavernous sinus
APB	Apex of the petrous bone
BA	Basilar artery
BS	Bony sinus
BSt	Brain stem
CA	Capsular artery(-ies)
CON	Canal of the optic nerve
CV	Cerebral vein
DA	Dawson's artery(-ies)
DP(ON)	Dura propria (optic nerve)
DR	Distal ring
ES	Ethmoid sinus
FL	Frontal lobe
FLa	Foramen lacerum
FO	Foramen ovale
FR	Foramen rotundum
FS	Frontal sinus
FSp	Foramen spinosum
FT	Fatty tissue
GPN	Greater (superficial) petrosal nerve
ILT	Inferolateral trunk
IVW	Inner venous wall
LM	Lilieqvist membrane
LPN	Lesser (superficial) petrosal nerve
LR	Lateral ring
LW	Lateral wall
MCA	Middle cerebral artery
MCF	Middle cranial fossa
MHT	Meningohypophyseal trunk
MM	Mucous membrane
MMA	Middle meningeal artery
OA	Ophthalmic artery
OT	Optic tract
OV	Ophthalmic vein
OVW	Outer venous wall
PB	Pituitary body
PCL	Petroclival ligament
PCoA	Posterior communicating artery
PCP	Posterior clinoid process
PICS	Posterior intercavernous sinus
PR	Proximal ring
PS	Pituitary stalk
PV	Petrosal vein
SCA	Superior cerebellar artery
SF	Sylvian fissure
SN(N)	Sympathetic nerve(s)
SOF	Superior orbital fissure
SPS	Superior petrosal sinus
SW	Sphenoid wall

TA	Tentorial artery	TM	Temporal muscle
TL	Temporal lobe	TTM	Tensor tympani muscle

Introduction

The anatomy of the cavernous sinus is extremely interesting but owing to its tridimensional character rather complex and difficult to understand. There is considerable difference between studying these anatomical relationships with the naked eye and studying them under the microscope. Surgically valid descriptions of the cavernous sinus anatomy have begun to appear only since magnification has become available. And again, examining a fresh cadaver specimen of the parasellar region with arterial and venous injection is vastly different to examination without injection.

Formalin-fixed preparations are almost useless for studying surgical anatomy since the relations between the individual structures may be significantly changed, distorted or even obliterated. It is only a fresh cadaver specimen with proper arterial and venous injection which can offer tridimensional relationships almost identical to those found in a living cavernous sinus. Yet this is still a far cry from a cavernous sinus with all its intricate venous and arterial pulsations in living human beings. However, by studying the anatomy of a fresh cavernous sinus specimen with good arterial and venous injection one can glean useful basic information on the anatomy of the cavernous sinus – information which is a sine qua non for one confronted in the operating theatre with another completely distorted anatomy of a diseased cavernous sinus.

A descriptive system utilizing the simplest geometric figure, the triangle, has been devised to facilitate orientation in the intricate maze of anatomical structures abounding in the parasellar region. The idea was to divide the said region into three subregions and ten surgical triangles defined by constant anatomical landmarks. Approaches through these triangles allow access to lesions in the cavernous sinus with minimum risk. The pertinent microsurgical anatomy, the system of nomenclature, and the possible application of surgical approaches to cavernous sinus lesions are presented. The author sincerely hopes that his modest contribution will be of value to all those who are willing to study the anatomy of the cavernous sinus and are ready to apply their knowledge of the subject derived herefrom.

1.1 Anatomy of the cavernous sinus

The macroscopic and microscopic anatomy of the parasellar skull base region has been increasingly investigated in recent years. As a result, the intracavernous anatomy of the nerves III through VI, the internal carotid artery (ICA) with its branches, and the related osseous structures and adjacent dural folds are well described [3, 12, 21, 23, 25, 33–37, 41, 42, 47, 51].

The surgical anatomy of the parasellar and adjacent skull base regions can be systematically divided into three subregions composed of ten triangles: (A) Parasellar subregion: (1) anteromedial triangle, (2) paramedial triangle, (3) oculomotor trigone, and (4) Parkinson's triangle; (B) Middle cranial fossa subregion: (1) anterolateral triangle, (2) lateral triangle, (3) posterolateral (Glasscock's) triangle, and (4) posteromedial (Kawase's triangle); and (C) Paraclival subregion: (1) inferomedial triangle and (2) inferolateral (trigeminal) triangle: (i) osseous portion and (ii) tentorial portion.

The margins of each triangle are based on the constant anatomical relationships of the osseous, dural, vascular, and neural structures located within the parasellar, middle cranial fossa and paraclival subregions. The purpose of this description of surgical triangles on the osseous borders and on the dural walls of the cavernous sinus (CS) is to define the boundaries of the CS and the windows in its walls through which different vascular and tumorous lesions in the CS can be reached and removed without damage to the vascular and/or neural structures of the CS.

Materials and methods

Parasellar regions from cadaveric skull base bone blocks (each consisting of the sphenoid bone, sella, CSs, medial portions of the petrous bones, clivus, and related structures) were examined using opton OPMI1 and opton OPMI6-CPC microscopes under 5–40 power. Specimens were obtained only from cadavers without historical or autopsy evidence of intracranial disease. Cranial nerves were divided as close to their exit from the brain stem as possible, with care taken to preserve dural folds, to retain accurate in situ anatomical relationships. After ligation of both supraclinoid ICAs and both posterior communicating arteries (PCoA), cannulation of the two proximal petrous ICAs was performed to allow colored acrylic injection of both carotid systems in each specimen. Colored acrylic injection of the venous compartments of the CS was performed through the superior and inferior petrosal sinuses. Photographs at appropriate stages of dissection were taken using a Canon A-1 35 mm camera.

Anatomical relationships

Osseous and dural structures

The most important bony landmarks on the medial aspect are the anterior clinoid process (ACP), the posterior clinoid process (PCP), and the lateral border of the clivus. On the dorsal aspect of the CS the most prominent structure is the anterior surface of the petrous bone whereas on the lateral aspect of the CS the most important landmarks are the superior orbital fissure (SOF), foramen rotundum, foramen ovale, and foramen spinosum.

The tentorium is attached to the petrous apex, to the PCP and ACP. These form a triangular field of dura referred to as the oculomotor trigone, at the lateral border of which the IIIrd and the IVth nerves enter the lateral wall of the CS. The margins of the oculomotor trigone include: (a) the anterior petroclinoid fold extending from the petrous apex to the ACP; (b) the posterior petroclinoid fold extending from the petrous apex to the PCP; and (c) the interclinoid fold extending between the ACP and the PCP [33]. Umansky and Nathan have previously reported that the lateral wall of the CS is consistently formed of two layers: the superficial, dense layer formed by the dura mater, and an inner reticular layer between which run the IIIrd, IVth and V1 nerves [51]. These authors also reported that in 40 % of their specimens the thin inner layer was incomplete, and often absent between the IIIrd nerve and V1, leaving a triangular opening onto the cavity of the CS. Medial to Meckel's cave, a layer of firm, fibrous connective tissue lies over the ICA, firmly fixing the ICA to the skull base. The well-formed anterior border of this fibrous bridge delineates the fixed portion of the ICA, which runs over the foramen lacerum from its mobile intracavernous portion. Peripheral to the Gasserian ganglion (GG) and along the lateral wall of the CS, the superficial dural layer can be separated from the inner reticular layer without entering the sinus. At the most anterior aspect of the CS, the two layers of dura separate to envelop the ACP and a part of the anterior loop of the ICA. The inner reticular layer runs inferior to the ACP and surrounds the anterior loop of the ICA forming its proximal ring which thus becomes the roof of the anterior CS, below and lateral to which are found the blood-filled venous trabeculated spaces medial to the ICA. The superficial dural layer continues over the superior surface of the ACP, tightly enveloping the ICA to form a separate ring referred to as the distal or dural ring. (According to this terminology, the adjectives "proximal" and "distal" describe the paraclinoid rings with respect to their location along the anterior loop of the ICA). It should be noted that a paraclinoid segment of the anterior loop of the ICA between the proximal and distal rings is extracavernous in location. The inner reticular layer continues medially, extending over the pituitary body, and inferiorly along the medial wall of the CS. The holes within the inner reticular layer provide for the passage of the intercavernous venous channels from the left to the right CS.

Oculomotor nerve

After exiting from the interpeduncular fossa, the IIIrd nerve runs in an anterolateral and slightly inferior direction in the anterior incisural space between the posterior cerebral artery and the superior cerebellar artery to enter the roof of the CS lateral to the PCP. At this point, the nerve acquires its own sheath of dura in the lateral portion of the anterior petroclinoid fold and continues anteriorly within the lateral wall of the CS.

Trochlear nerve

The IVth nerve exits from the dorsal surface of the midbrain just below the inferior colliculus at the level of the superior medullary velum. In the cerebello-mesence-phalic fissure the nerve curves anteriorly around the lateral aspect of both the tectum and tegmentum in the quadrigeminal and ambiens cisterns, then continues in the antero-latero-inferior direction to enter the inferior surface of the tentorial edge lateral to the cerebral peduncle. It then runs anteriorly for several millimeters in a groove on the inferior surface of the tentorium before becoming completely encased in the dural canal. After entering the tentorium, the IVth nerve continues anteriorly, following the margin of the anterior petroclinoid fold to enter the lateral wall of the CS where running inferior and lateral to the IIIrd nerve it is embedded between two dural layers.

Trigeminal nerve

After arising from the lateral pons, the motor and sensory roots of the Vth nerve run in an anterior and lateral direction through the middle incisural space of the posterior cranial fossa superior to the petrous apex to enter the subarachnoid and dural outpouching known as Meckel's cave. Several millimeters superior and posterior to the entry of the Vth nerve into Meckel's cave is the dural entry point of the petrosal vein into the SPS. Ventro-medial to Meckel's cave at the petrous apex is the lateral loop of the ICA, which runs over the foramen lacerum. A previous study indicated that the bone separating the dura of Meckel's cave and the ICA was absent in 68 % of specimens [12]. In these cases, the GG was separated from the ICA by a layer of fibrous connective tissue. The greater superficial petrosal nerve (composed of pre-ganglionic parasympathetic fibers), after exiting from its hiatus in the anterior side of the petrous bone, runs anteriorly and epidurally over the floor of the middle cranial fossa to join the Vth nerve. As the fascicles of the Vth nerve lose their arachnoid covering, they coalesce to form the GG which gives off V1, V2, and V3. V3 continues inferiorly, laterally, and slightly anteriorly to leave the middle cranial fossa via the foramen ovale several millimeters lateral to the foramen lacerum. V2 runs anteriorly and slightly inferiorly between the two dural layers to leave the middle cranial fossa through the foramen rotundum. Here, V2 forms the inferolateral margin of the CS. Before entering the SOF, V1 runs anteriorly between two dural layers of the lateral wall of the CS where it is located inferolateral to the IVth nerve and superomedial to V2.

Abducens nerve

The VIth nerve extends anterosuperiorly through the prepontine cistern after leaving the anterior pontomedullary sulcus. The nerve pierces the dura overlying the basilar venous plexus of the clivus. The fascicles of the VIth nerve are sometimes divided, forming several individual nerve bundles at the entry point into the clival dura. The length of the nerve within Dorello's canal is somewhat variable, depending on its dural entry point. After entering Dorello's canal, the VIth nerve continues superiorly and slightly medially in close apposition to the bone, forming the cortex of the distal clivus. It then runs anteriorly and slightly medially beneath the fibrous petroclinoid ligament, close to the base of the PCP, to enter the venous spaces of the CS, lateral to both the proximal segment of the medial loop of the ICA and the horizontal portion of the ICA, and medial to V1. A small spicule of bone is commonly found along the apex of the petrous bone at the lateral end of the petroclinoid ligament, with the nerve coursing immediately medial to this bony prominence and lateral to the ICA to enter the CS; it continues laterally as it courses anteriorly within the venous trabeculae of the CS. In some cases the petroclinoid ligament is completely calcified, forming a foramen through which the nerve enters the CS.

Internal carotid artery

After running through the bony carotid canal and over the foramen lacerum, ventro-medial to Meckel's cave, the ICA in its sheath of sympathetic fibers courses beneath the previously described fibrous connective tissue bridge to enter the posterior portion of the CS, lateral to the base of the PCP. Usually, the cavernous ICA has three major groups of branches [12, 42], the largest, most proximal and most constant of these branches being the meningo-hypophyseal trunk (MHT), which extends medially from the medial loop of the cavernous ICA, to divide into the tentorial artery, the dorso-meningeal artery, and the inferior hypophyseal artery. A few millimeters distally, the artery of the inferior CS (also called the infero-lateral trunk (ILT) or the lateral main stem artery) arises from the inferolateral aspect of the horizontal segment of the ICA. After coursing superior to the VIth nerve, it gives off branches to the lateral dural wall of the CS and to the adjacent cranial nerves.

The horizontal segment of the intracavernous ICA then runs medially and superiorly to form a U-turn referred to as the anterior loop. In 30 % of specimens the distal horizontal segment of the ICA has been found to give rise to McConnor's capsullar arteries, making them the least consistent branches of the cavernous ICA [12, 41]. The inferior and anterior capsullar branches have been described as supplying the floor and the roof of the sella, respectively. In approximately 8 % of cases the ophthalmic artery arises from the intracavernous (extradural) ICA [12]. As described previously, the inner layer of the dura forms the proximal dural ring providing the barrier separating the intracavernous ICA from its extracavernous paraclinoid portion. Four to six millimeters distally, the dura surrounds the ICA to form the distal dural ring separating the paraclinoid portion of the anterior loop from the intradural supraclinoid ICA. The supraclinoid ICA enters the subarachnoid space lateral to the optic nerve (ON) and medial to the ACP.

Intracavernous relationships

The cranial nerves III, IV, and V1 continue anteriorly between the superficial and the reticular dural layers forming the lateral wall of the CS to enter the SOF. Throughout the posterior portion of the CS these nerves maintain a constant relationship to each other with regard to the superior – inferior orientation, although the course of the IVth nerve, inferior to the IIIrd nerve and superior to V1, has been shown in a previous study to be somewhat more variable anteriorly within the lateral wall of the CS [23]. However, 5–7 mm posterior to the bony margin of the SOF, the IVth nerve runs superiorly along the lateral aspects of the IIIrd nerve, crossing over the IIIrd at this point; it continues anteriorly, now superior and slightly lateral to the IIIrd nerve, to enter the SOF.

The IVth nerve runs inferior to the petroclinoid ligament and then enters the posterior CS maintaining its direction throughout the lateral wall of the CS lateral to the cavernous ICA and adjacent to the medial aspect of V1. Sympathetic fibers, running with the ICA, coalesce into discrete fiber bundles, which leave the ICA to join the VIth nerve for several millimeters before crossing over to join V1, with which they run peripherally to provide sympathetic innervation in the corresponding trigeminal territory. As the VIth nerve continues anteriorly, it assumes a slightly more inferior location within the CS in relation to V1, so that, at the level of the SOF, the VIth nerve is both medial and inferior to V1.

In addition to the VIth nerve, sympathetic fibers, venous trabecular channels, and the intracavernous ICA, variable amounts of fatty connective tissue are also found throughout the CS. Other potential venous tributaries include the superior and inferior ophthalmic veins, the superior and inferior petrosal sinuses, the sphenoparietal sinus, cortical veins, veins of the pterygoid plexus, via the foramen ovale, and the basilar venous plexus.

The relationships of the intracavernous structures, predominantly of the ICA and venous compartments to the bony sinuses and to the sella, will be discussed in detail.

1.2 The surgical triangles of the cavernous sinus

The constant anatomical relationships of the dural, osseous, neural and vascular structures of the parasellar skull base region permit the organization of the relevant anatomy into a series of ten triangular windows, each with its particular surgical significance in skull base lesions. One of these triangles has been further subdivided into osseous and tentorial portions. These ten triangles have been grouped into three subregions (the parasellar, the middle cranial fossa, and the paraclival one). Conceptually, the two-dimensional triangles can be expanded into three-dimensional spatial figures to form a series of ten tetrahedrons, each containing specific dural, osseous and neuro-vascular structures. For the sake of simplicity and consistency, however, the term »triangle« will be retained throughout this book to include the three-dimensional extension of each triangle with its specific contents.

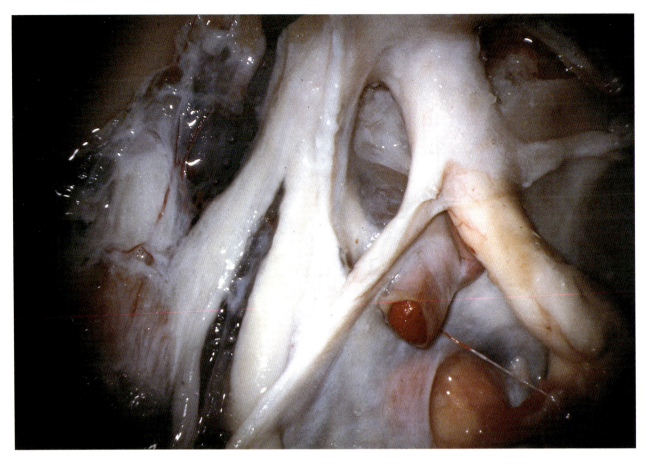

Fig. 1. A fresh cadaver specimen with red acrylic injected into the arteries and blue transparent acrylic injected into the venous compartments. The ACP and the outer dural layer of the lateral wall of the CS have been removed. The anteromedial triangle is bordered medially by the ON covered with the dura propria, laterally by the IIIrd nerve covered with the fibrous tissue of the proximal ring, and by the dura extending from the entry point of the IIIrd nerve to the ON. On the floor of the anteromedial triangle the anterior loop of the ICA, covered by venous blood and by a thin fibrous layer, is seen. Anterior to the anterior loop of the ICA is the mucous membrane of the sphenoid sinus. Posterior to the anterior loop of the ICA, fibrous tissue is seen between the dura and the IIIrd nerve

Parasellar subregion

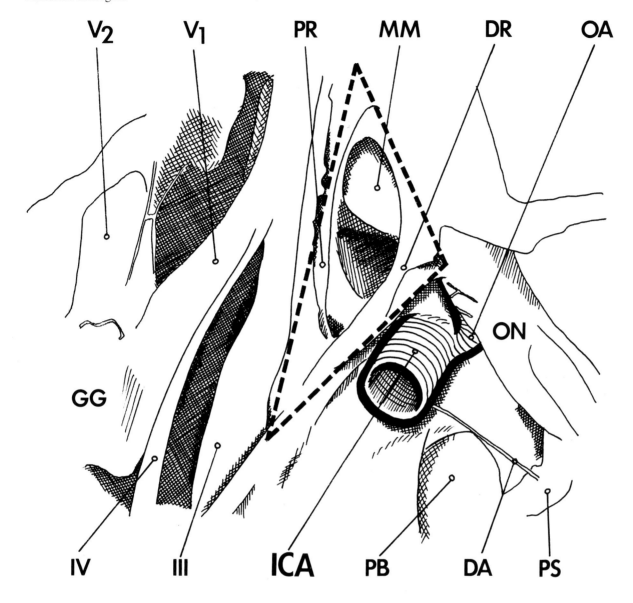

Anteromedial triangle

The sides of this triangle include: the lateral aspects of the ON confined within the optic canal (medial border); the medial aspects of the IIIrd nerve within the sheath of dura entering the SOF (lateral border); and the dura extending between the dural entry point of the IIIrd nerve and the ON (posterior border), which forms the dural ring around the paraclinoid ICA [8, 9] (Fig 1). Exposure of the anteromedial triangle requires complete extradural removal of the ACP. Impor-

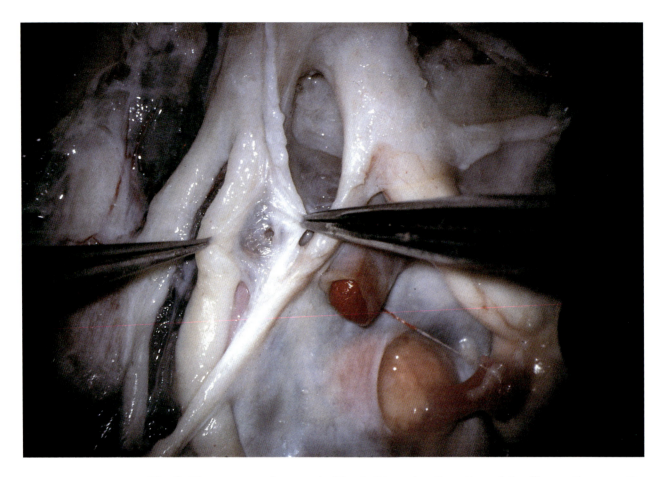

Fig. 2. The same specimen as in Fig. 1. Step-wise dissection of the fibrous tissue on the medial aspect of the IIIrd nerve has been performed. It can be clearly seen that the fibrous tissue layer running from the dura along the medial aspect of the IIIrd nerve is strong and that it divides the extracavernous from the intracavernous area of the anteromedial triangle

tant structures within the anteromedial triangle include: (i) the distal horizontal segment of the intracavernous ICA, the anterior loop of the ICA, (ii) the venous trabecular channels of the anteromedial portion of the CS, and (iii) a thin layer of fibrous connective tissue continuous with that surrounding the anterior loop of the ICA thus forming the proximal dural ring of the paraclinoid ICA. The anterome-

V₂   V₁   OV   PR   MM   DR   ON

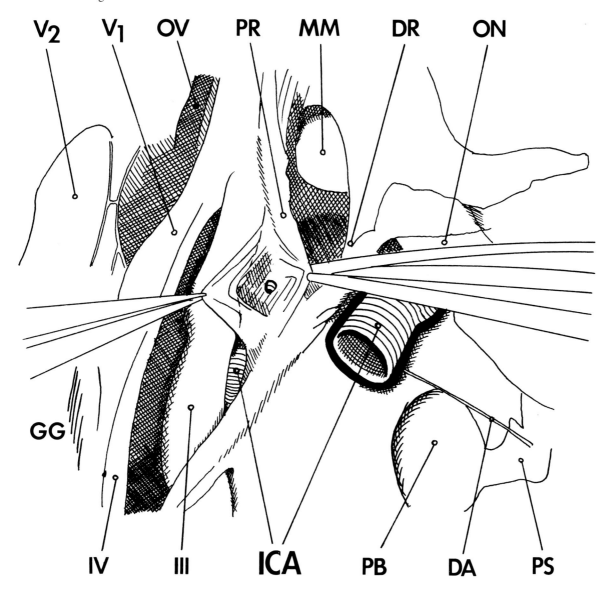

GG

IV   III   **ICA**   PB   DA   PS

dial triangle therefore includes the extradural space occupied by the ACP as well
as the anteromedial portion of the CS. These two adjacent regions are separated
by the connective tissue of the proximal dural ring extending toward the PCP along
the lateral aspect of the sella.

The anteromedial triangle of the **left** CS is shown in Figs. 1–5.

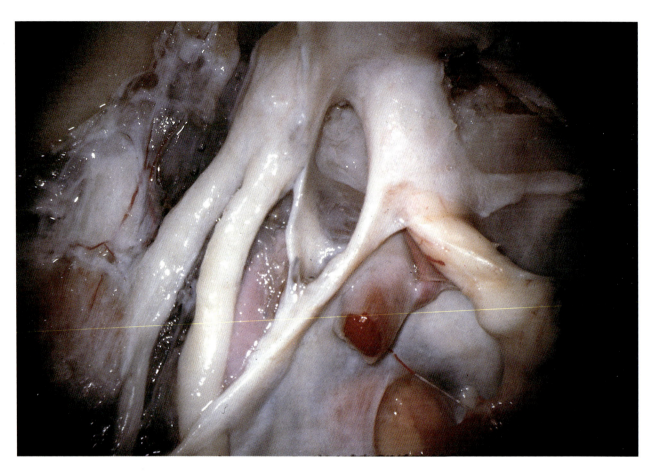

Fig. 3. The proximal ring dividing the extracavernous from the intracavernous area of the anteromedial triangle, also covers the most anterior segment of the anterior loop of the ICA. It can be seen that lateral to the proximal ring, part of the horizontal portion of the ICA is visible through the anteromedial triangle. This segment of the ICA is imbedded in "venous blood" as is seen underneath the IIIrd nerve

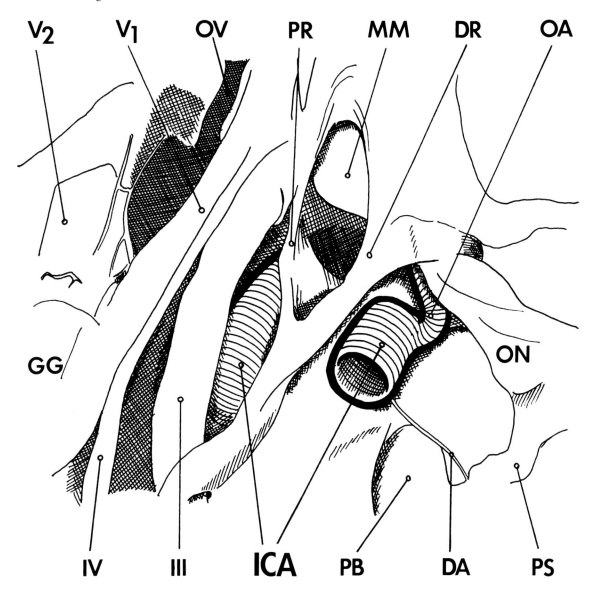

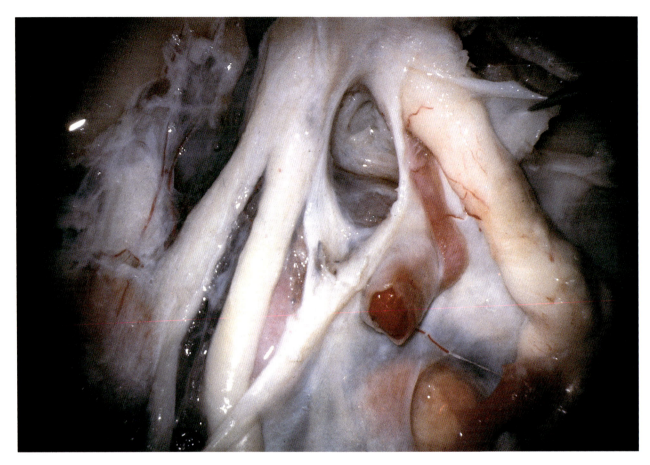

Fig. 4. The anteromedial triangle can be further enlarged by cutting the dura propria along
the longitudinal axis of the ON. By dissecting the ON from the dura propria the nerve can
be displaced transversely to its longitudinal axis, whereby space is gained. By displacing
the ON medially, the ophthalmic artery is fully exposed. In this manner, the medial aspect
of the distal dural ring of the ICA can be reached and cut off entirely

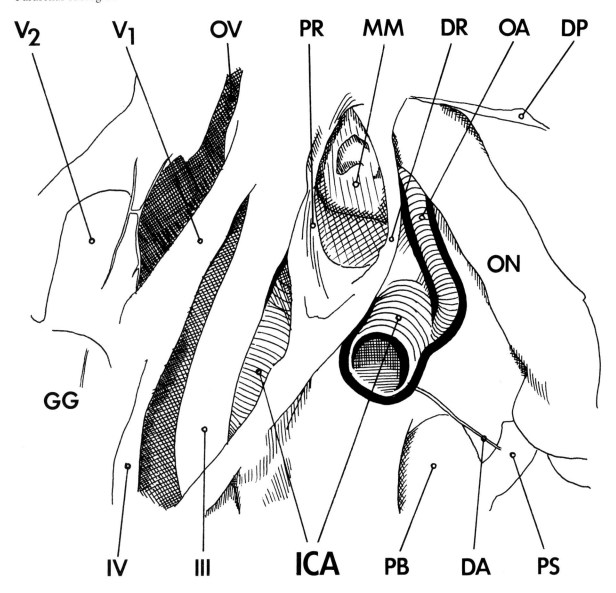

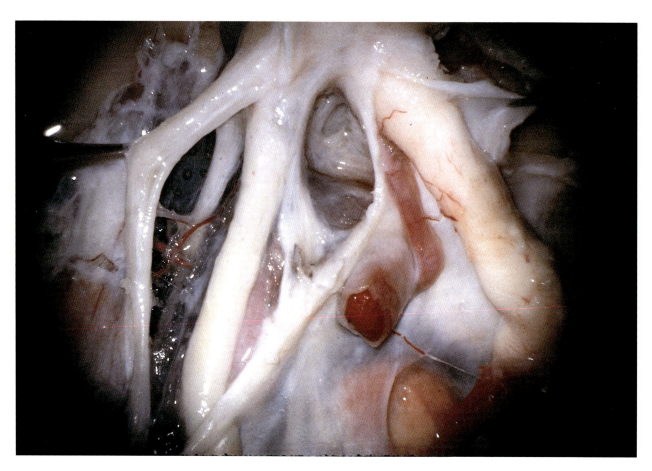

Fig. 5. The anteromedial triangle can also be enlarged laterally. Retraction of V1, the IVth and/or the IIIrd nerve(s) offers a much better access to the horizontal portion of the ICA. The ILT running over the VIth nerve can be identified either from the lateral side of the IIIrd nerve through the paramedial triangle, as shown, or from the medial side of the IIIrd nerve through the anteromedial triangle (not shown)

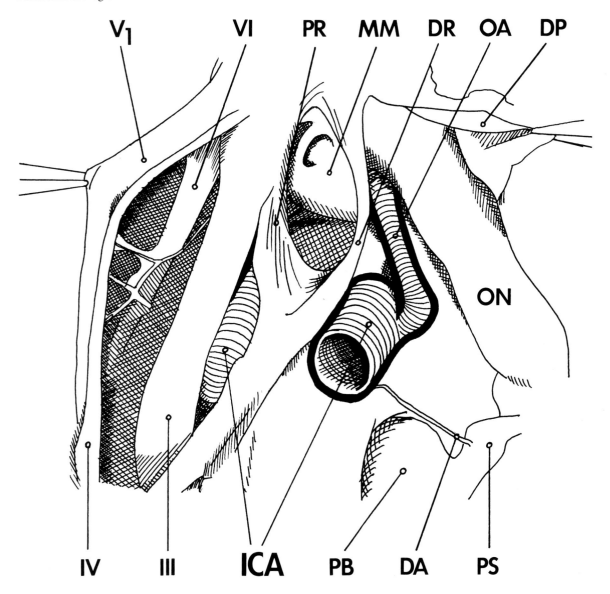

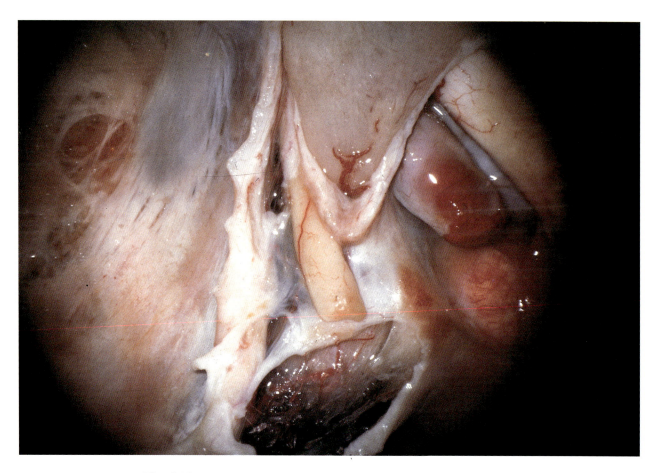

Fig. 6. The IIIrd nerve running along the lateral aspect of the ACP forms the medial border of the paramedial triangle. It can be seen that the nerve is covered by a thick fibrous dural layer on both the medial and the proximal side, and by a thin transparent reticular layer on the inferior aspect facing the CS. The lateral border of the paramedial triangle is formed by the IVth nerve. The dura between the entry points of nerves IV and III forms the base of the paramedial triangle and is part of the lateral border of the oculomotor trigone

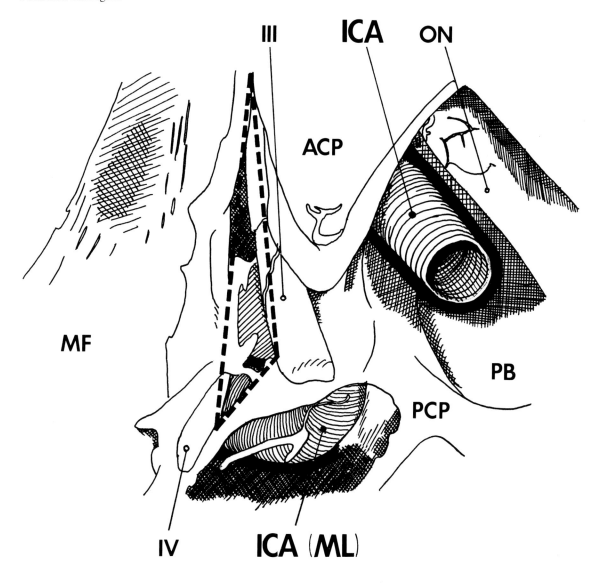

Paramedial triangle

The lateral aspect of the IIIrd nerve (medial border), the medial aspect of the IVth nerve (lateral border), and the dura extending between the dural entry points of nerves III and IV (posterior border) (Fig. 6). It should be noted that just posterior to the SOF, the IVth nerve courses on the lateral and superior aspects of the IIIrd nerve, before both nerves enter the SOF (Figs. 8–10). Therefore, the anterior apex of the paramedial triangle is formed by the point at which the IVth nerve crosses

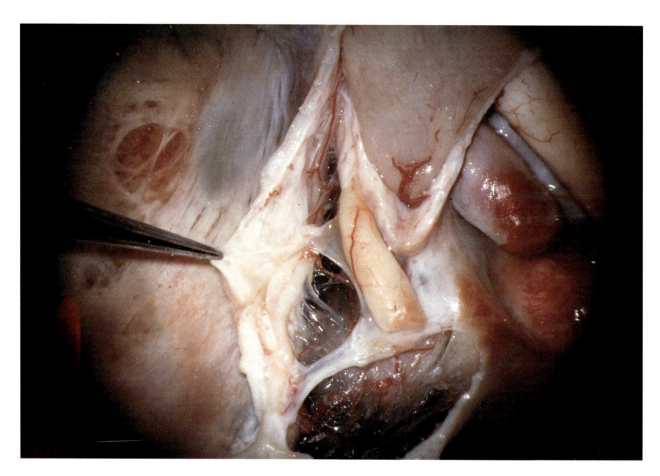

Fig. 7. The paramedial triangle has been widened a little. The reticular layer lying on the inferior aspect of the IIIrd nerve extends over the IVth nerve. The inferior aspect of the IVth nerve has almost no covering. In this particular specimen, the IIIrd nerve is separated from the IVth by a thin reticular layer of the lateral wall of the CS. Note that the arterial blood supply of nerves III and IV is provided mainly by the ILT. Part of the medial loop of the ICA is visible through the transparent injection in the venous compartments

over the IIIrd nerve. Structures of significance within the paramedial triangle include: the horizontal segment of the intracavernous ICA, the branches of the ILT, the venous trabecular channels of the CS, sympathetic fibers, the dural roof of the CS, and, in some cases, the medial loop of the ICA, the MHT and the proximal intracavernous segment of the VIth nerve.

The paramedial triangle of the **left** CS is shown in Figs. 6–10.

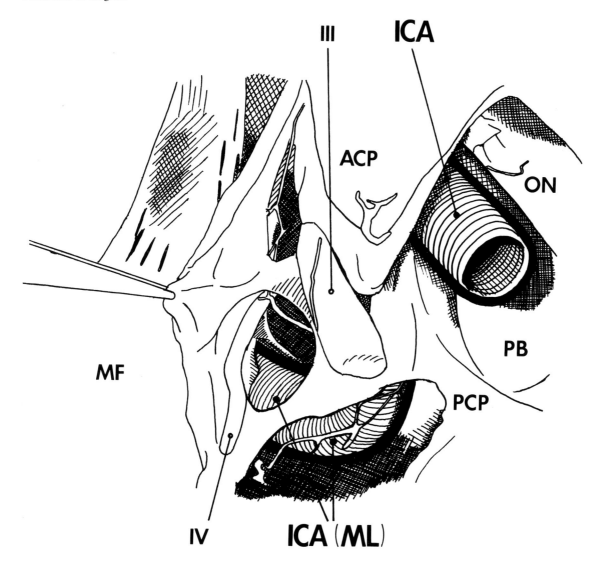

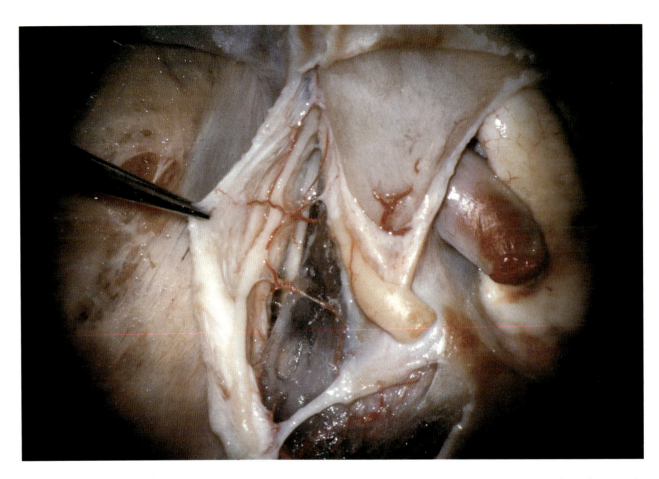

Fig. 8. The paramedial triangle is enlarged by retraction of the lateral wall of the CS. In this manner, V1 and the VIth nerve as well as the larger part of the medial loop of the ICA are visualized. Note the rich arterial blood supply of the nerves and huge amount of "venous blood" in this area

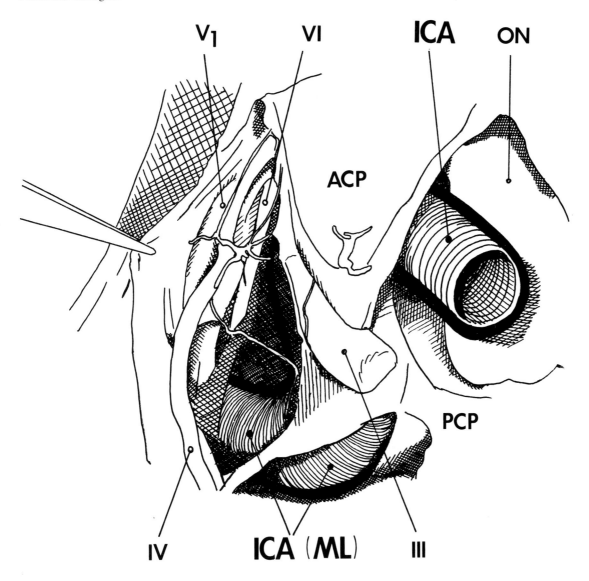

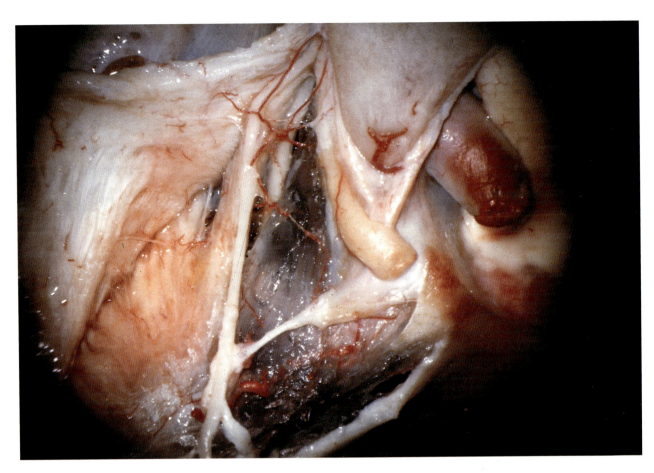

Fig. 9. By lateral retraction of the outer layer of the lateral wall of the CS, the paramedial triangle is widened. In this way, the VIth nerve in the CS is seen crossing the ICA and the course of the nerve lateral to the horizontal segment of the ICA is visualized. By cutting the base of the paramedial triangle, the inferomedial triangle can be easily reached. If the MHT is not visible through the paramedial triangle, it can be reached by further dissection from the paramedial into the inferomedial triangle. The GG is shown lateral to the IVth nerve

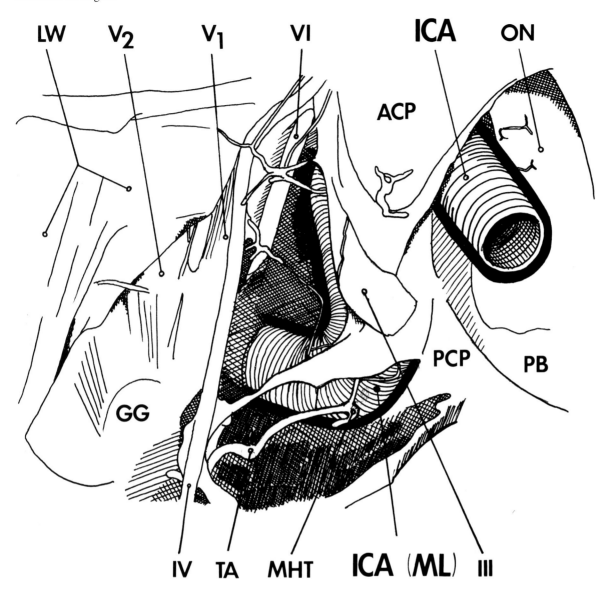

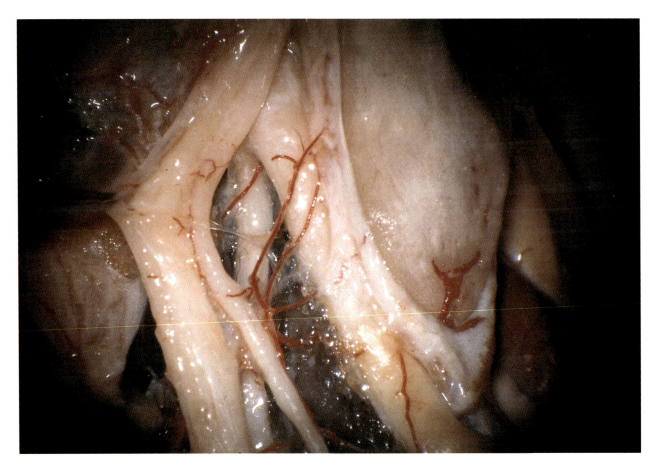

Fig. 10. The anterior part of the paramedial triangle is shown under higher magnification. Its most important feature is that the IVth nerve and V1 run over the IIIrd nerve before they enter the SOF. Deep in the center of this corner, the VIth nerve is seen embedded in "venous blood"

Oculomotor trigone

The triangular area of the oculomotor trigone, described previously [33], is located between the folds of the dura running between the ACP and the PCP, and medially with the fold of the dura running from the PCP to the ACP. This triangle is situated posterior to the base of the paramedial and anteromedial triangles, and anterolateral to the inferomedial triangle. On the lateral border of the oculomotor triangle lie the entry points of the IIIrd and the IVth nerves into the lateral wall of the CS.

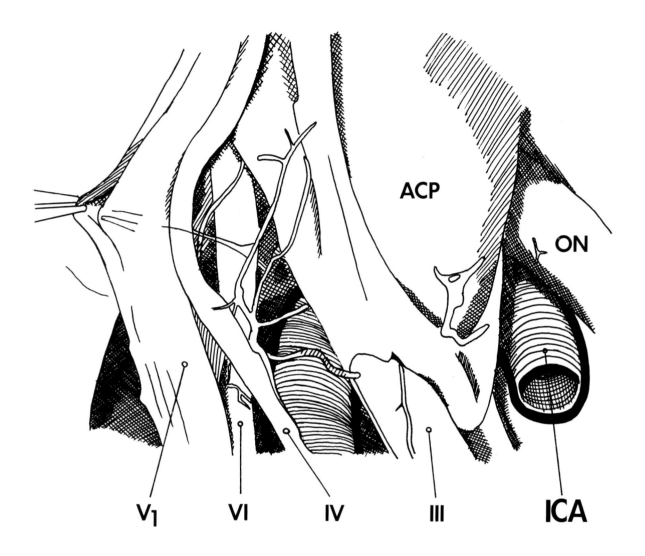

Through the oculomotor triangle, the tip of the medial loop of the ICA, the medial aspect of the medial loop of the ICA, and the medial aspect of the horizontal segment of the ICA can be reached. In surgery involving the anteromedial, paramedial or inferomedial triangle, the oculomotor trigone is also usually opened.

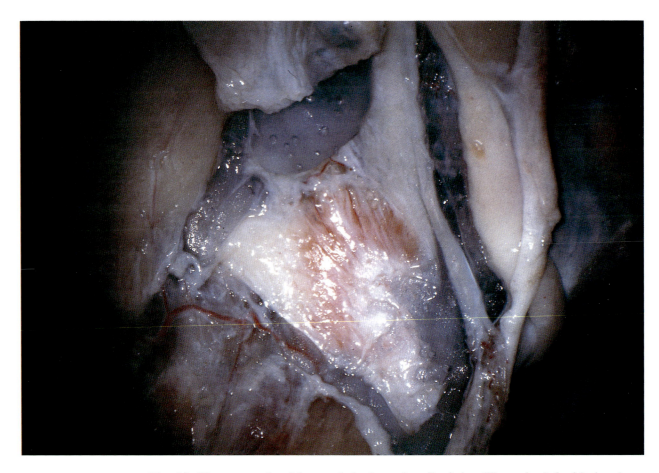

Fig. 11. The outer, dural layer of the lateral wall of the CS on the left side has been removed. "Venous blood" is abundant. The amount of "venous blood" in the CS can be estimated and its outflow toward the SPS is well visualized. The IVth nerve is in very close proximity to the medial aspect of V1. In this particular case Parkinson's triangle lies rather posteriorly and is bordered by the IVth nerve medially, the GG and the Vth nerve laterally and the dura at the base

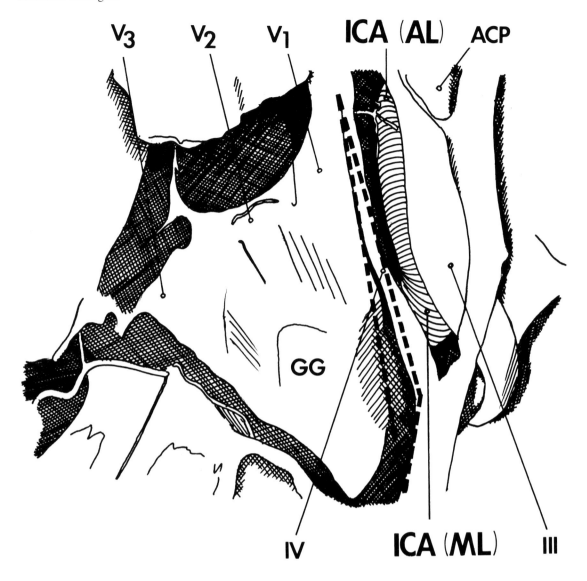

V₃ V₂ V₁ ICA (AL) ACP

GG

IV ICA (ML) III

Parkinson's triangle

Parkinson's triangle is delineated by the IVth nerve (medial border), the medial aspect of V1 (lateral border), and the dura between these two nerves posteriorly (posterior border). Through Parkinson's triangle the following structures can be seen: the medial loop of the cavernous ICA with, in most cases, the MHT, venous trabecular channels, the proximal and midcavernous segments of the VIth nerve, sympathetic fibers, and the dura forming the superior portion of the lateral wall of

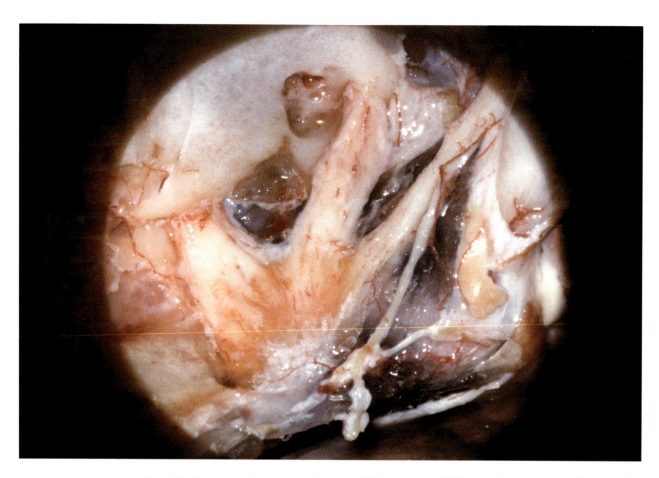

Fig. 12. Since, in this preparation, the IVth nerve and V1 have been separated, only the anterior segment of the former nerve is attached to the latter one. Through the triangle "venous blood" is seen to run posteriorly over the Vth nerve into the SPS

the CS. It should be noted that the region of the incomplete, and often absent, inner reticular layer between the IIIrd nerve and V1, described by Umansky and Nathan, corresponds to the region of the dura of the CS over the paramedial and Parkinson's triangles [51].

Parkinson's triangle of the **left** CS is shown in Figs. 11–13; Fig. 14 shows Parkinson's triangle of the **right** CS.

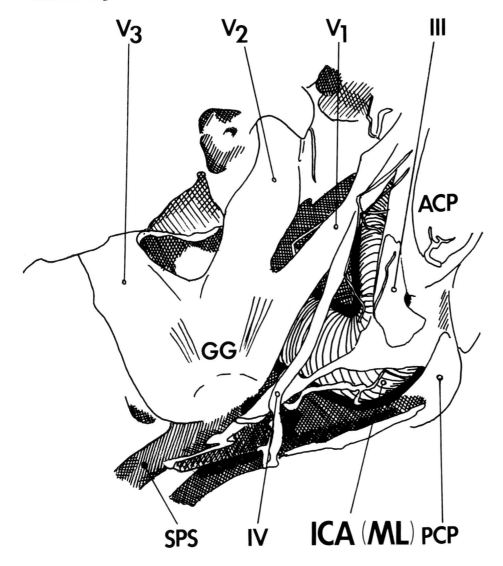

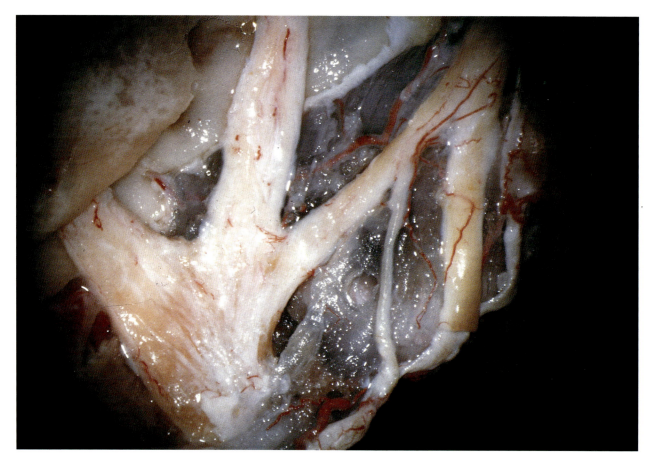

Fig. 13. Through the widened Parkinson's triangle good access is gained to the MHT, the ICA and the VIth nerve. A large segment of the ICA running from the lateral loop above the foramen lacerum toward the medial loop adjacent to the PCP can be safely exposed through this triangle

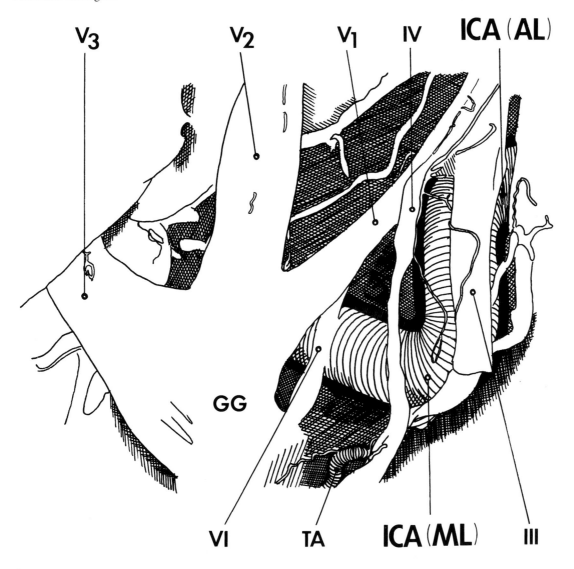

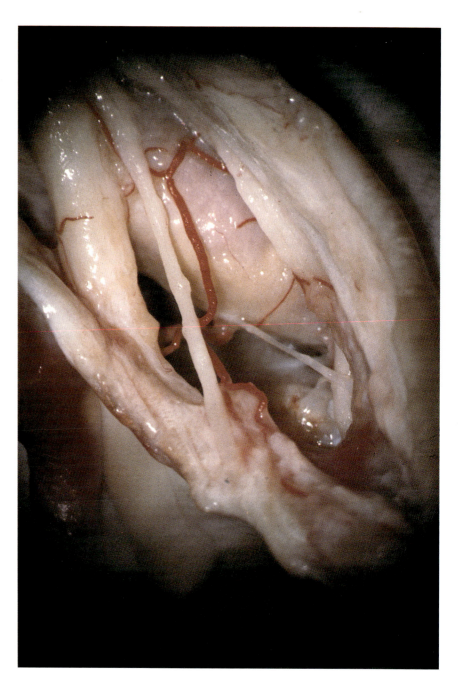

Fig. 14. Through Parkinson's triangle the medial loop of the ICA, the MHT, the ILT and the VIth nerve are seen. The entire medial loop of the ICA is visualized from both the medial and lateral sides. On the medial side of Parkinson's triangle the paramedial triangle is wide open. The VIth nerve on the lateral side is covered by the GG and V1

III   IV   ILT   ICA(ML)

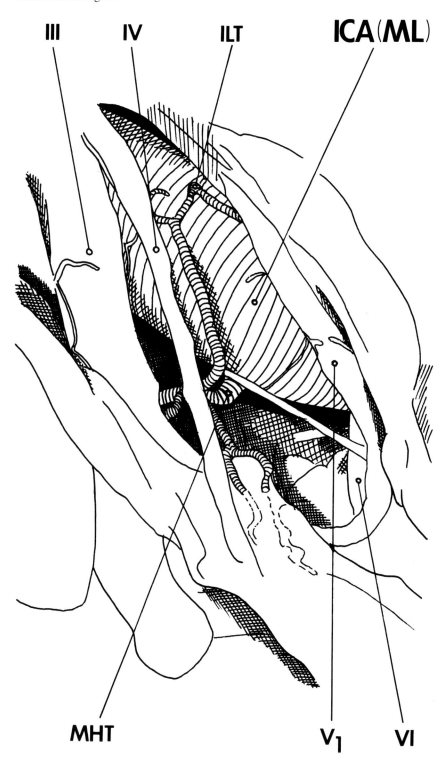

MHT   V₁   VI

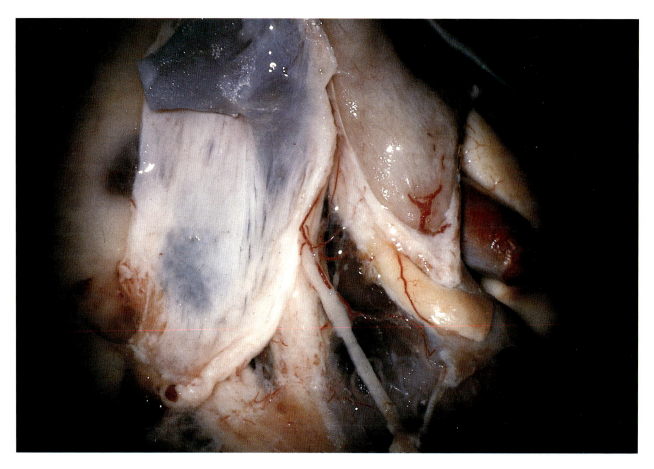

Fig. 15. In the anterior area of the anterolateral triangle a huge vein enters the lateral wall of the CS. The intense blue color of the lateral wall of the CS indicates that there is abundant blood between its layers

Middle cranial fossa subregion

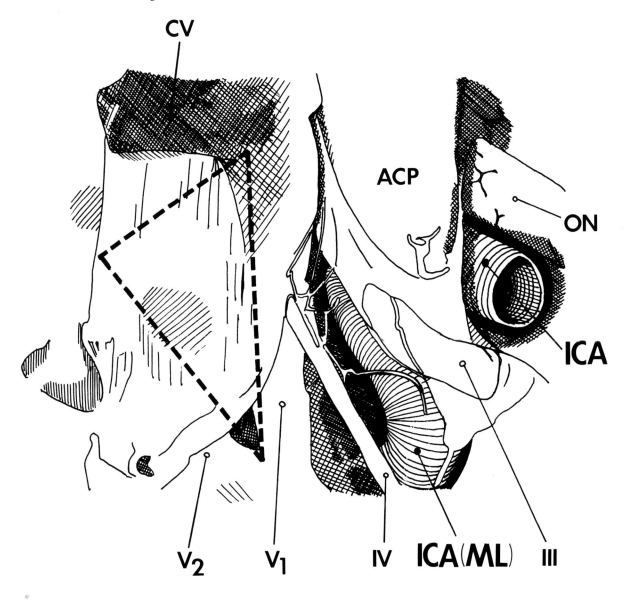

Anterolateral triangle

The lateral edge of V1 (medial border), the medial edge of V2 (lateral border), and the anterolateral wall of the bony middle cranial fossa (anterior border). Through the anterolateral triangle the following structures are seen: the inferolateral aspect of the distal horizontal portion of the cavernous ICA, the dura and the anterior bony floor of the middle cranial fossa, the venous trabecular channels of the inferolateral CS, and the dura forming the inferior portion of the lateral wall of

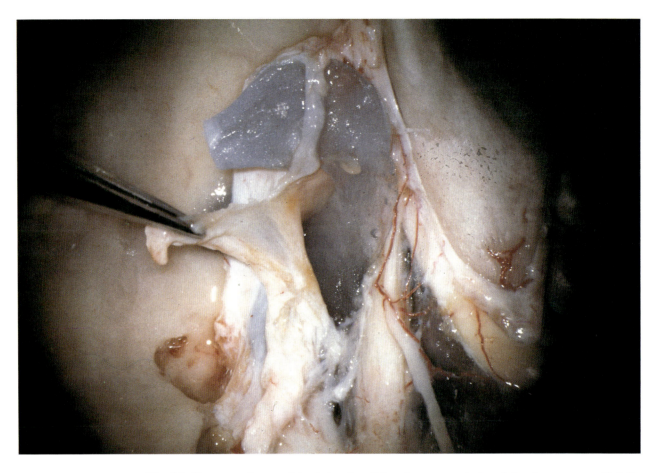

Fig. 16. The outer layer of the lateral wall has been resected and the "venous pool" fully exposed between the two layers of the lateral wall of the CS

the CS. Within this triangle the distal intracavernous portion of the VIth nerve is inferolateral to V1 as it courses anteroinferiorly toward the SOF.

The anterolateral triangle of the **left** CS is shown in Figs. 15–20.

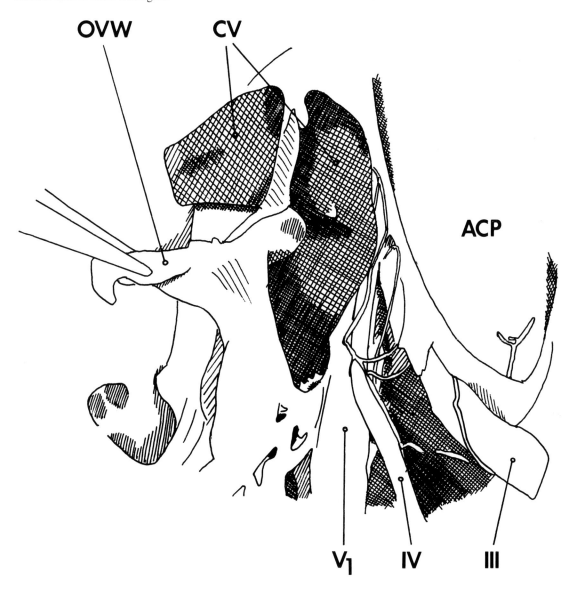

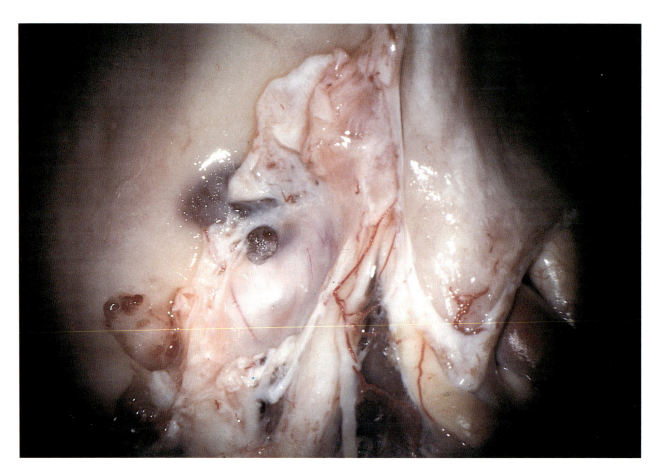

Fig. 17. The inner layer of the lateral wall in the area of the anterolateral triangle lying over V1 and V2 is visualized after removal of the "venous pool". At the most anterior point of the anterolateral triangle the inflow of "venous blood" from the vein into the CS is seen. Due to the engorged vein, in the lateral wall of the CS, V1 is displaced medially

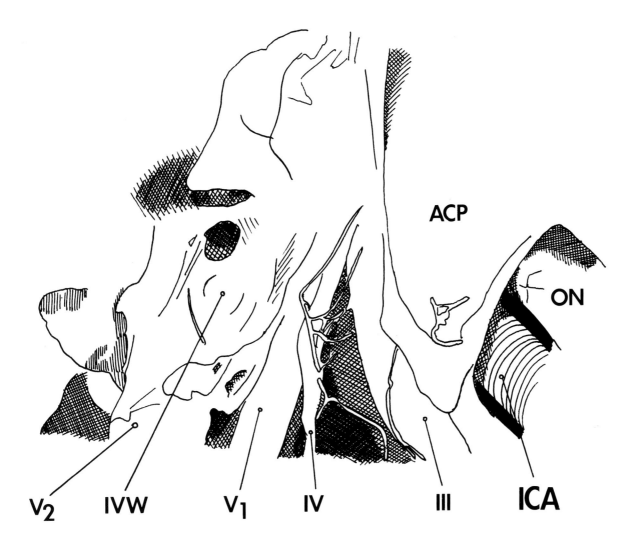

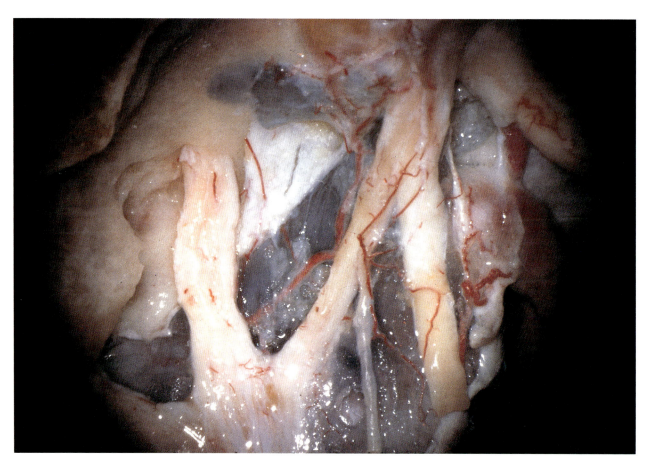

Fig. 18. The inner layer of the lateral wall of the CS lying over V1 and V2 has been removed. In this manner the anterolateral triangle is fully exposed. In the anterior part of the anterolateral triangle the fibrous-dural tissue over the bone is intact. The numerous arterial branches supplying the nerves and surrounding structures, as well as "venous blood" in the CS, are shown

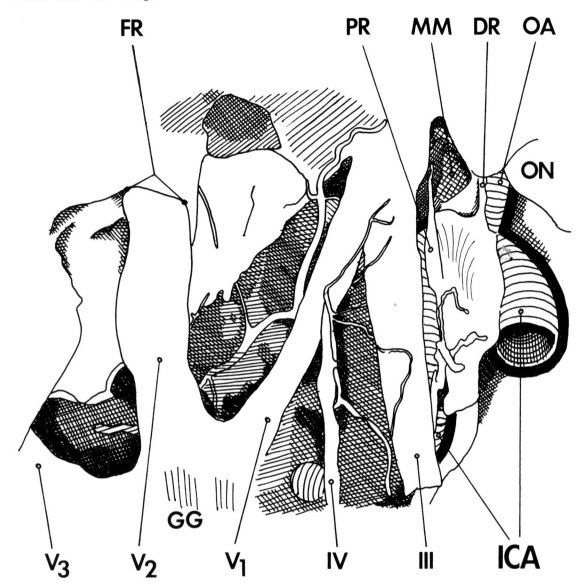

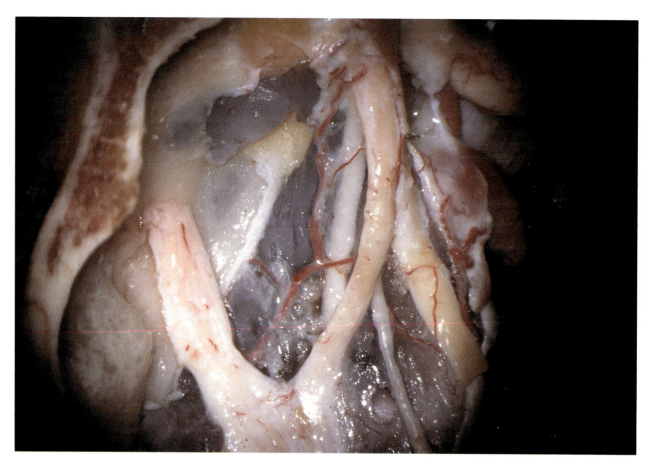

Fig. 19. The entire anterolateral triangle is shown from its apex at the GG to its base at the bone of the middle fossa between the SOF and the foramen rotundum. At the front part of the anterolateral triangle "venous blood" is seen covering the fatty tissue usually found in this region. Slight retraction of V1 toward the medial side exposes the VIth nerve. The "venous pool" in the sinus as well as the arterial branches supplying the nerves are shown

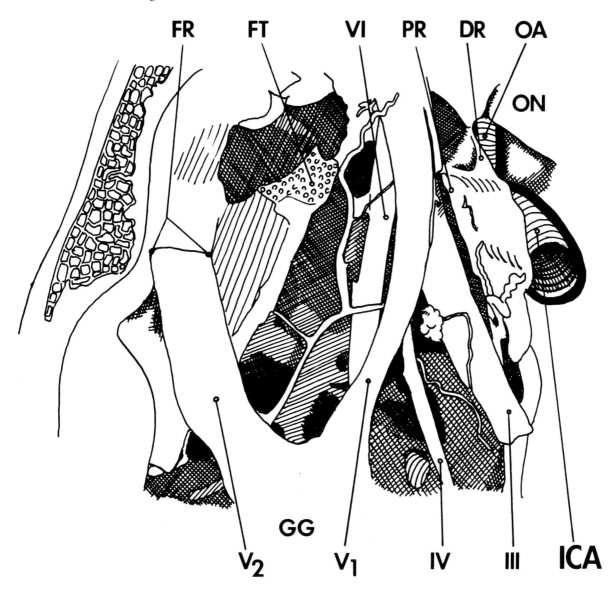

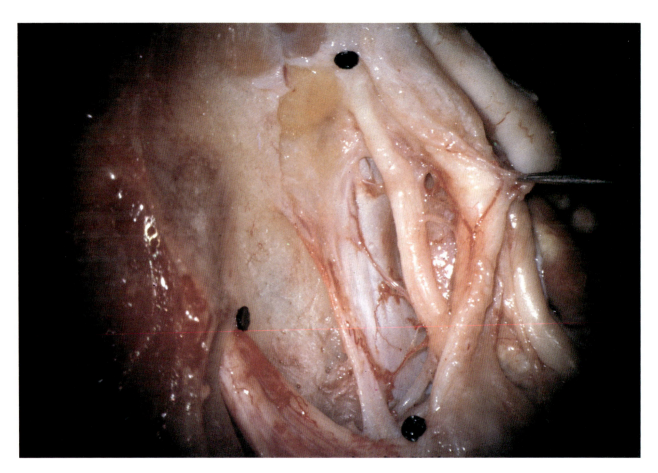

Fig. 20. Through this triangle a large segment of the VIth nerve can be seen. For better visualization of the VIth nerve, the ICA and the sympathetic fibers running from the ICA to the VIth nerve and hence to V1, it is necessary to retract V1 medially. The fibrous covering of the bone is the direct continuation of the dura which runs from the apex of the petrous bone, forms the lateral ring around the ICA medial to the foramen lacerum, and proceeds further anteriorly to cover the bone. The fatty tissue at the anteromedial corner of the anterolateral triangle is most probably a continuation of the fatty tissue from the orbit. The 3 black dots are for better visualization of the triangle

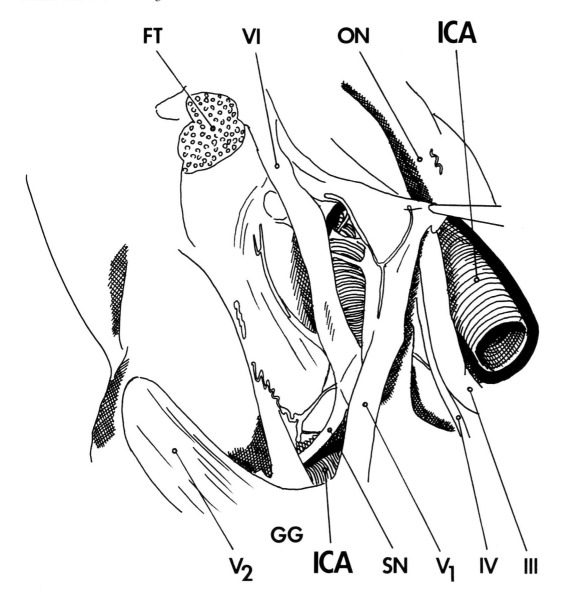

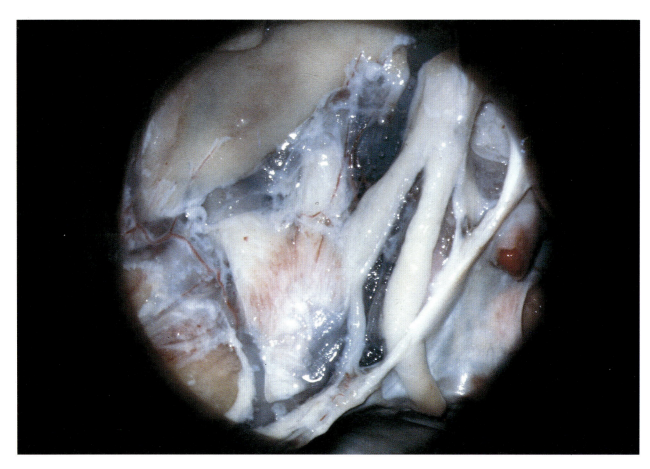

Fig. 21. The lateral wall of the CS and the dura over the bone have been removed. Of all the triangles (anteromedial, paramedial, Parkinson's, anterolateral) shown in this figure, the lateral triangle, confined between V2, V3 and the bone between the foramen rotundum and foramen ovale, is the smallest one. The whole area of the lateral triangle is filled with "venous blood"

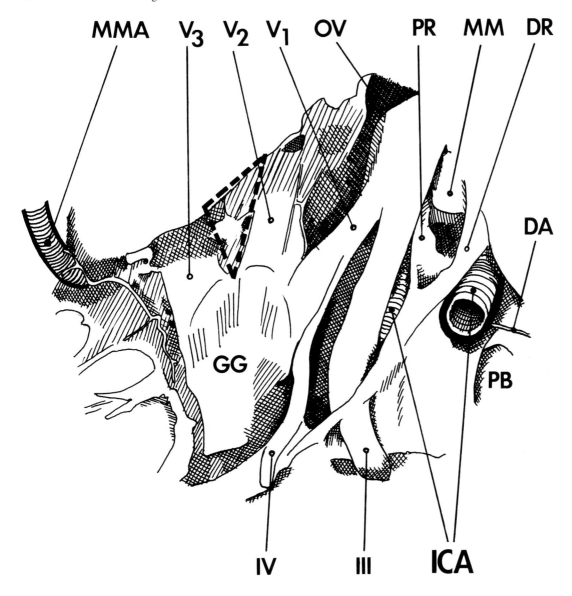

Lateral triangle

The lateral edge of V2 (anteromedial border), the anterior edge of V3 (posterior border), and the lateral wall of the bony middle cranial fossa (lateral wall). Through this triangle the anterior and lateral aspects of the lateral loop of the ICA, as well as the sympathetic fibers on the ICA, can be reached. Owing to the short course of V3 and the proximity of the GG, slight retraction of V3 and V2 is possible without endangering the function of these two branches. By laterally drilling the bone of the middle fossa additional space is gained for a better lateral approach.

The lateral triangle of the **left** CS is shown in Figs. 21–25.

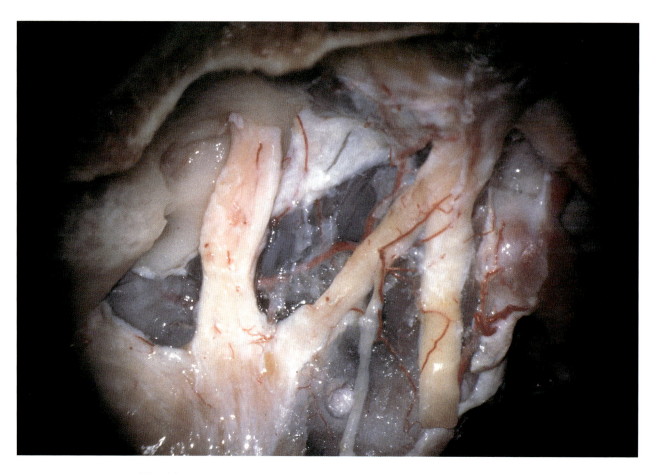

Fig. 22. The lateral triangle is much smaller than the anterolateral triangle. It is completely filled with "venous blood". Through the transparent blue venous injection, the arterial branch is visible. Note that V3 is much shorter than V2 and that the GG is much closer to the foramen ovale than to the foramen rotundum

FO   FR   PR MM DR OA

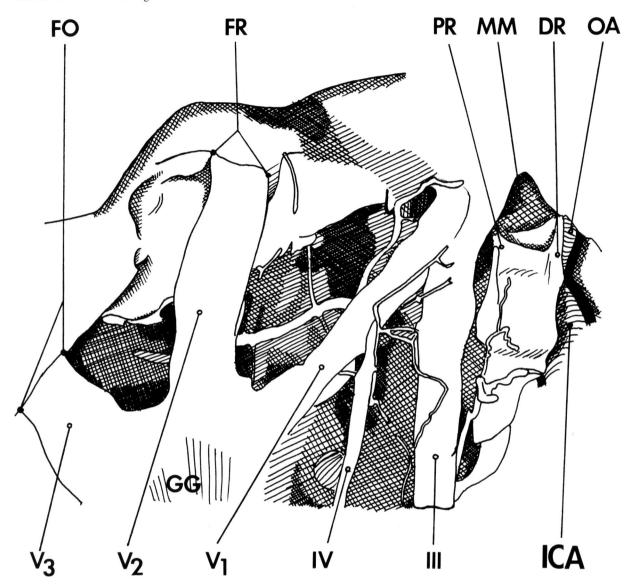

GG

V₃   V₂   V₁   IV   III   ICA

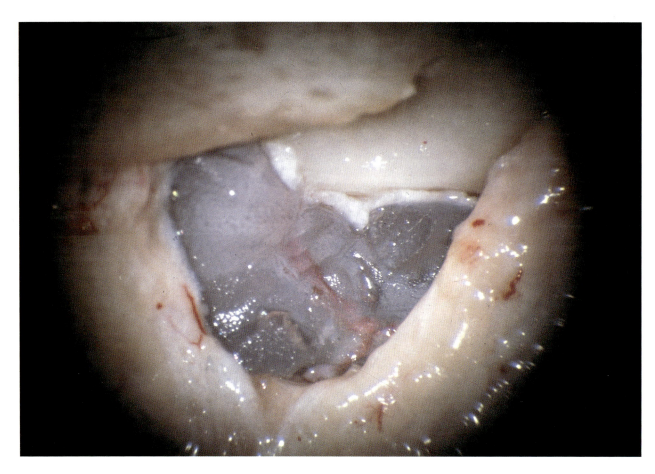

Fig. 23. The lateral triangle is shown under higher magnification. The only possibility of enlarging this triangle is by drilling the bone in a lateral direction. In order to gain better access to the space below the GG, the bone is ground laterally. Through the grey blue transparent venous injection the arterial branch is seen

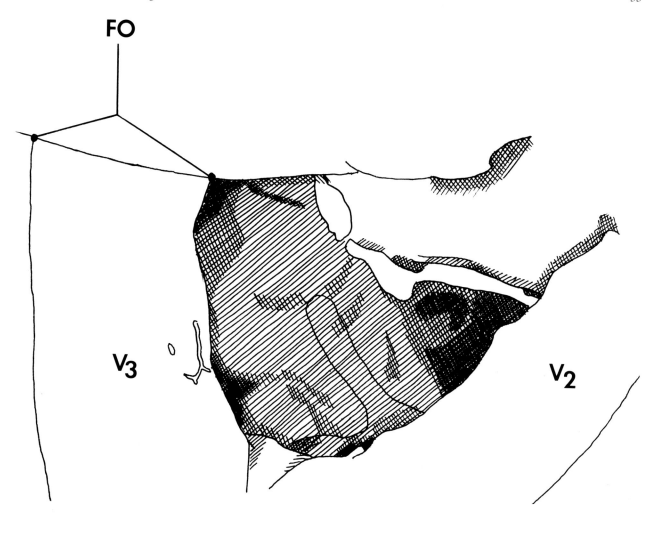

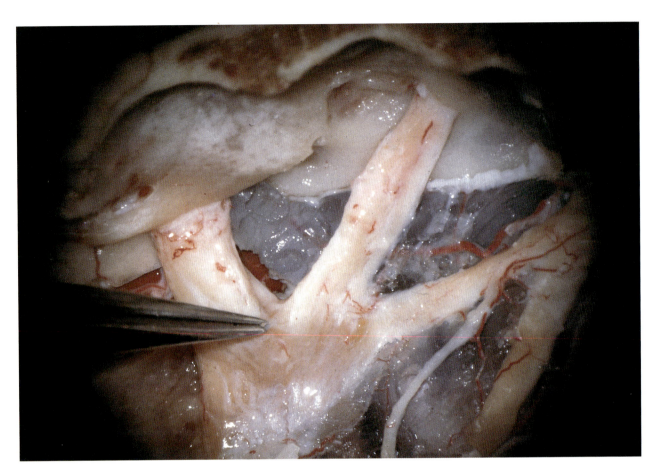

Fig. 24. After removal of "venous blood" and slight retraction of the GG, the lateral loop of the ICA can be reached. Thus, the lateral triangle is very important for it gives a safe access to the lateral loop of the ICA

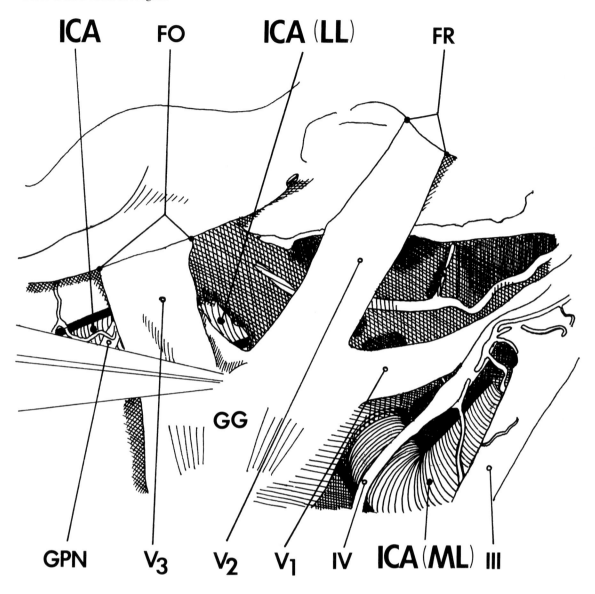

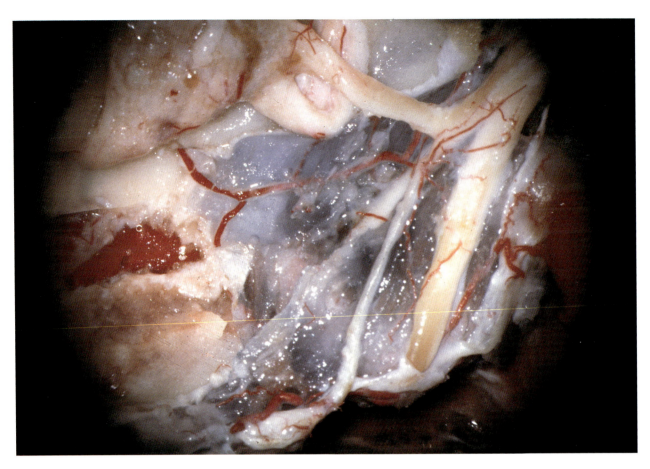

Fig. 25. The Vth nerve together with the GG is elevated thereby exposing the lateral loop. In this figure, the entire course of the ICA from the foramen lacerum to the PCP, that is, from the lateral to the medial loop, can be traced. Since during surgery the Vth nerve cannot be elevated, different segments of the ICA must be approached through different triangles

ICA (PL) V₃ V₂ V₁ VI PR DR OA

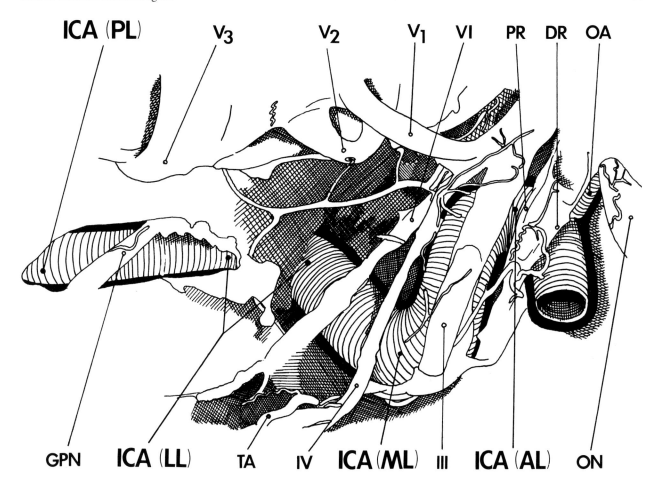

GPN ICA (LL) TA IV ICA (ML) III ICA (AL) ON

Posterolateral (Glasscock's) triangle

The greater superficial petrosal nerve (medial border), the posterior aspect of the GG and V3 (anterior border), and the line between the foramen spinosum and the arcuate eminence of the petrous bone (posterior border) [10]. Through this triangle the following important structures are seen: the posterior loop of the ICA, the proximal portion of the lateral loop of the ICA covered by the anterior aspect of the petrous apex forming the posteromedial floor of the middle cranial fossa,

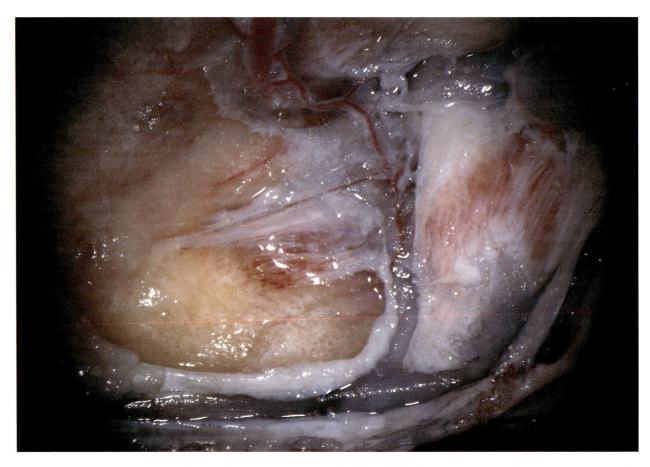

Fig. 26. From the posterior part of the left middle fossa the dura has been removed and the Vth nerve and the GG have been exposed. The venous outflow from the CS on each side of the Vth nerve is in a posterior direction toward the SPS. The anterior aspect of the apex of the petrous bone is exposed posterior to the GG and the Vth nerve. On the lateral side of the sphenopetrous fissure, the middle meningeal artery is seen together with its branch. Lateral to the sphenopetrous fissure and to the greater petrosal nerve is the posterolateral triangle. On the medial side of the sphenopetrous fissure and greater petrosal nerve is the posteromedial triangle

the labyrinthine branch of the middle meningeal artery coursing parallel to the greater superficial petrosal nerve, the greater and lesser superficial petrosal nerves and the tensor tympani muscle and the Eustachian tube separated from the ICA by a 1–2 mm thick bone wall. It should be noted that within this region the structures coursing nearly along the parasagittal plane maintain a parallel relationship to each other.

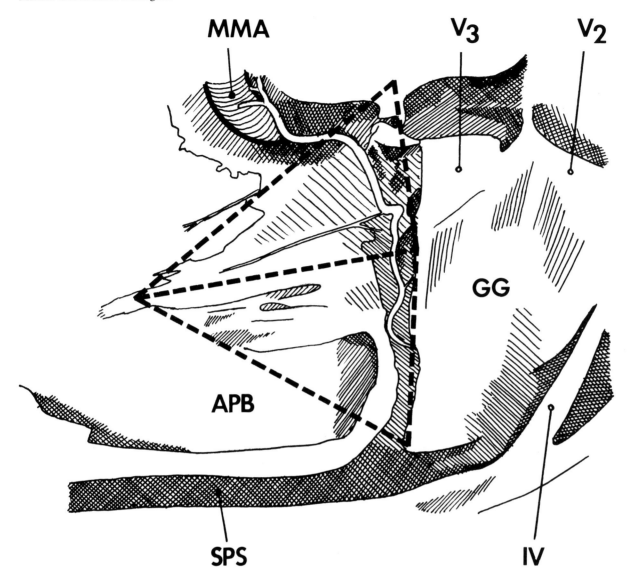

Posteromedial (Kawase's) triangle

The posterior border of the GG (anterior border), the sphenopetrosal groove with the greater superficial petrosal nerve (lateral border), the line connecting the hiatus of the greater superficial petrosal nerve and the posterior aspect of the Vth nerve where it crosses the crest of the petrous apex (posterior border) [17, 18]. The posteromedial triangle includes the dura, the bone of the petrous apex, and a portion of the SPS. The importance of this triangle is twofold. By drilling the

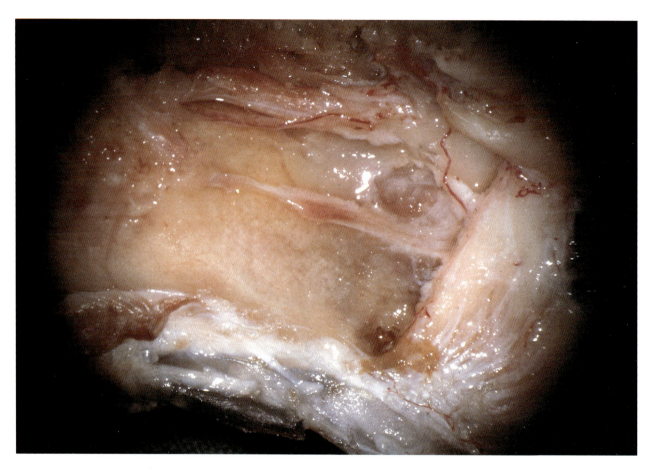

Fig. 27. Posterior to the GG and lateral to the sphenopetrous fissure and greater petrosal nerve, the thin bony layer covering the petrous ICA has been partially removed and the ICA exposed. On the lateral and dorsal aspects of the ICA canal in the petrous bone, the lesser petrosal nerve and the tensor tympani muscle are seen. Medial to the greater petrosal nerve and posterior to the trigeminal nerve, the posteromedial triangle is located. Medial to the apex of the posteromedial triangle, the SPS running parallel to the greater petrosal nerve but in an anteroposterior direction, is seen

bone behind the GG and the Vth nerve, the posterior fossa can be entered, the region behind the Vth nerve explored, and the clivus reached. By more extensive drilling of the apex of the petrous bone, the anterior portion of the inner auditory canal can also be exposed. The second important point is that by drilling the

VII   LPN   TTM   **ICA**   V₃

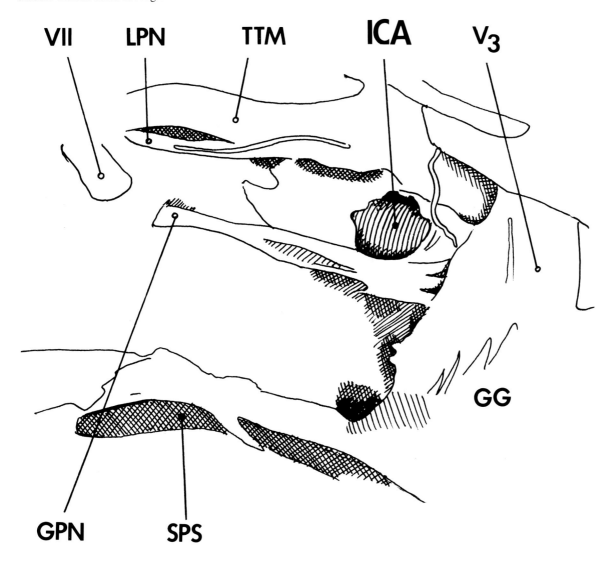

GPN   SPS   GG

petrous apex, the medial aspect of the posterior loop of the ICA can be well visualized and prepared for temporary clipping, and/or grafting.

The posterolateral and posteromedial triangles of the **left** CS are shown in Figs. 26–30.

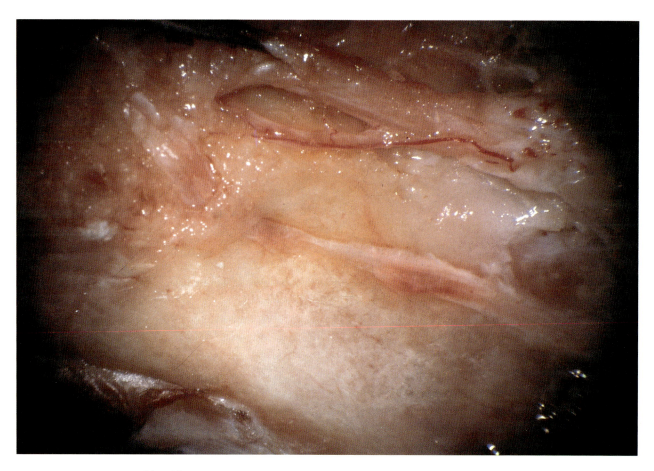

Fig. 28. Lateral to the posterolateral triangle the tensor tympani muscle and the lesser petrosal nerve are seen. The petrous portion of the ICA in the carotid canal has been partially unroofed. In this specimen the petrous segment of the ICA is situated lateral to the sphenopetrous fissure and the greater petrosal nerve medial to the ICA. The geniculate ganglion of the facial nerve has been unroofed and the exit of the greater petrosal nerve from the VIIth nerve is seen. Medial to the sphenopetrous fissure and the greater petrosal nerve, the area of the posteromedial triangle is seen

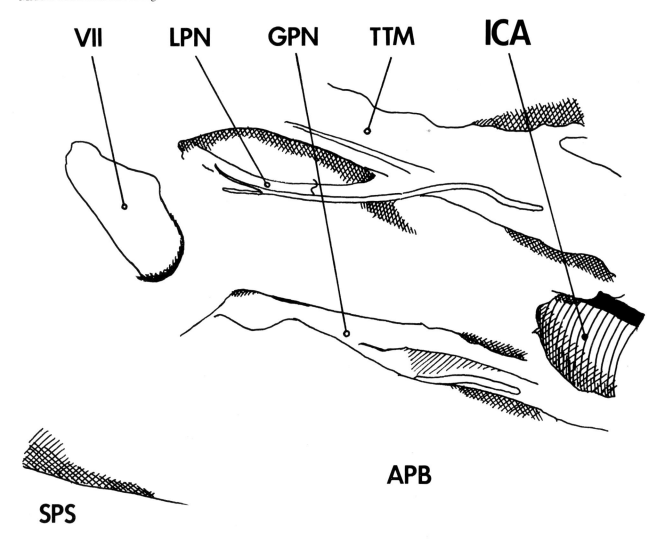

VII   LPN   GPN   TTM   ICA

SPS

APB

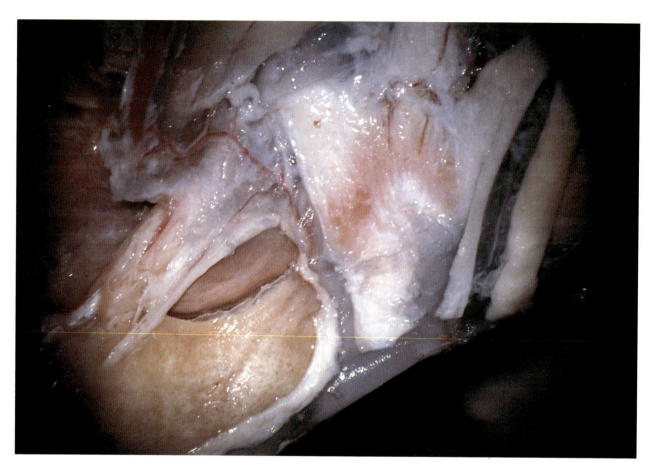

Fig. 29. The posterior loop of the ICA in the petrous bone has been unroofed. In this specimen, the ICA is located medial to the sphenopetrous fissure, and the greater petrosal nerve is almost on the lateral aspect of the posterior loop of the ICA. The tensor tympani muscle and the Eustachian tube are seen. The rest of the petrous apex medial to the posterior loop of the ICA forms the posteromedial triangle. The Vth nerve with the GG and all three branches, is surrounded with venous injection showing that the venous outflow is toward the SPS

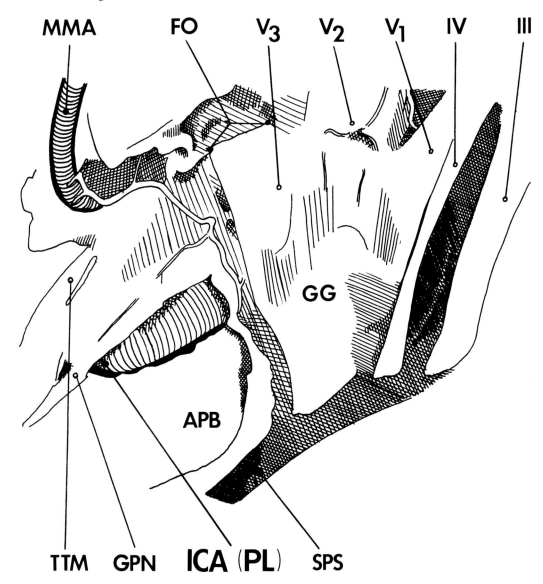

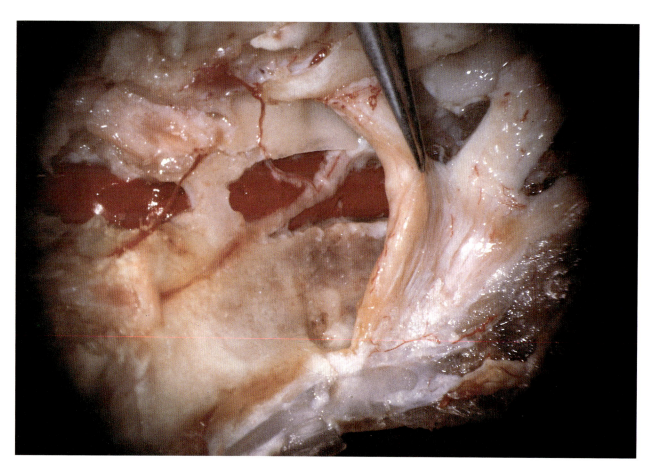

Fig. 30. The carotid canal has been unroofed and the injected ICA is shown. The tensor tympani muscle with the Eustachian tube is on the lateral aspect of the ICA; the lesser and the greater petrosal nerves cross the ICA. The greater petrosal nerve runs over the ICA toward the foramen lacerum, and the ICA runs underneath V3 and the GG where it forms the lateral loop. The anterior surface of the apex of the petrous bone representing the posteromedial triangle posterior to the GG and medial to the Vth nerve, to the sphenopetrous fissure and to the ICA, is still in place. The SPS is in continuity with venous compartments over the Vth nerve and in Parkinson's triangle

ICA (PL)   ICA (LL)   FR   V₃   V₂   V₁

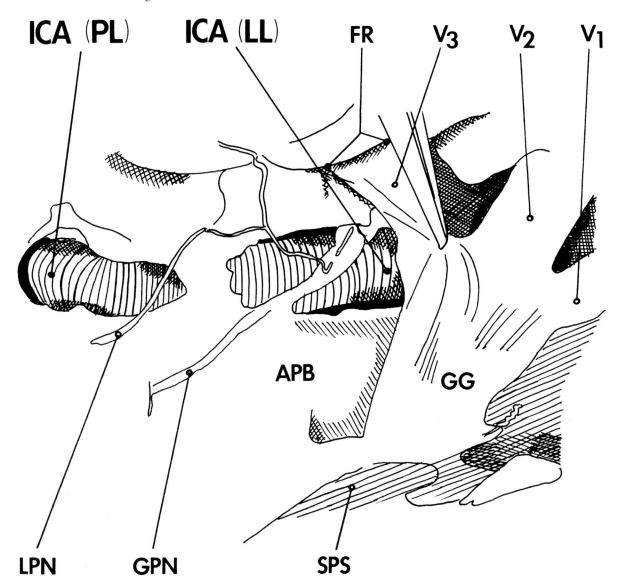

LPN   GPN   SPS   APB   GG

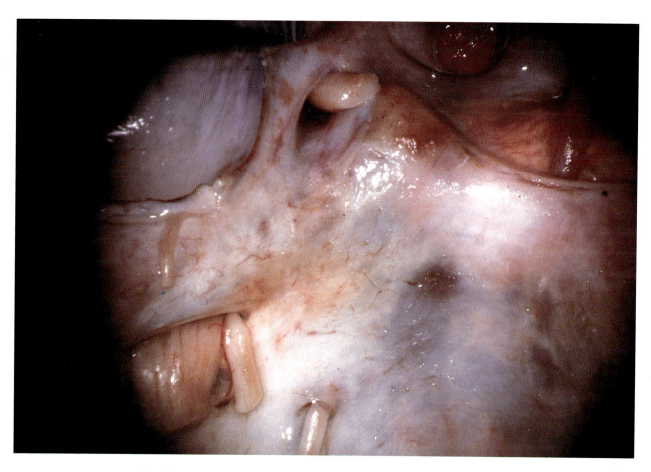

Fig. 31. The left paraclival area with the inferomedial triangle can be seen. The proximal border of the triangle is defined by the posterior dural fold running from the entry point of the IVth nerve on the inferior aspect of the tentorium toward the tip of the PCP. The medial border is the line between the entry point of the VIth nerve and the tip of the PCP, and the lateral border of the triangle is the line connecting the entry points of the VIth and the IVth nerves. The superior border of the inferomedial triangle is at the same time the dorsal border of the oculomotor trigone in which the large entry site of the IIIrd nerve is seen. Through the thin dura on the clivus, the intense blue color of the venous injection is seen

Paraclival subregion

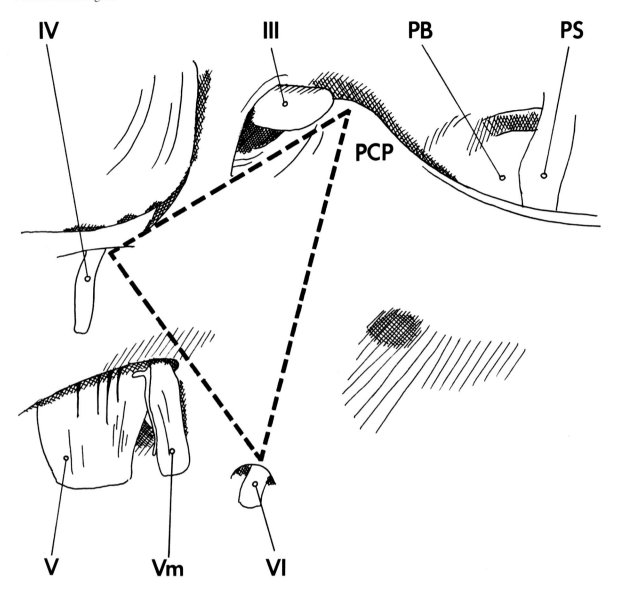

Inferomedial triangle

The triangle is formed by the tip of the PCP (medial point), the dural entry point of the IVth nerve into the tentorium (laterosuperior point), and the dural entry point of the VIth nerve into Dorello's canal (lateroinferior point). The structures of importance within this triangle include: the basilar venous plexus and its overlying dura, the dura forming the posterior wall of the CS, the posterior petroclinoid fold, the segment of the VIth nerve within Dorello's canal under the petroclinoid

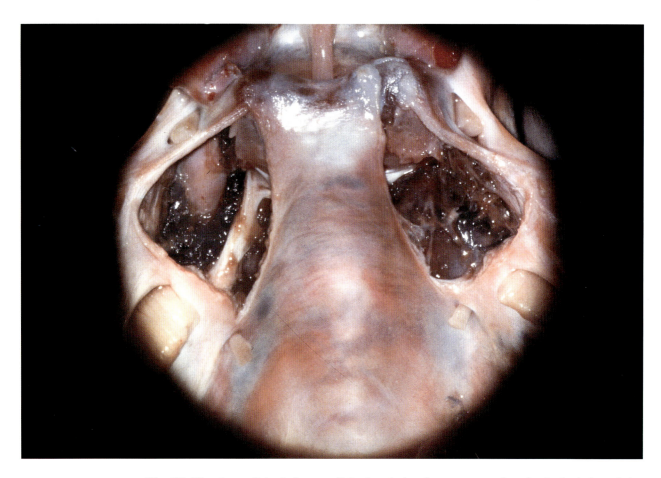

Fig. 32. The dura of the inferomedial triangle has been removed on both the left and the right sides. On the right side, the venous injection is left in place. Beside the venous injection in the medial corner of the right inferomedial triangle, the dorsal aspect of the PCP is seen. In the left inferomedial triangle, however, part of the venous injection has been removed and the petroclinoid ligament and the posterior aspect of the medial loop of the ICA are exposed. The left and right VIth nerves can be seen intradurally and not yet extradurally in the CS. Both IIIrd nerves, both IVth nerves, and both Vth nerves are seen intradurally. In the sagittal line anteriorly, the pituitary stalk can be seen

ligament extending toward the lateral aspect of the ICA, the petroclinoid ligament, and the dorsal meningeal branch of the MHT.

The inferomedial triangle of the **left** CS is shown in Figs. 31–35.

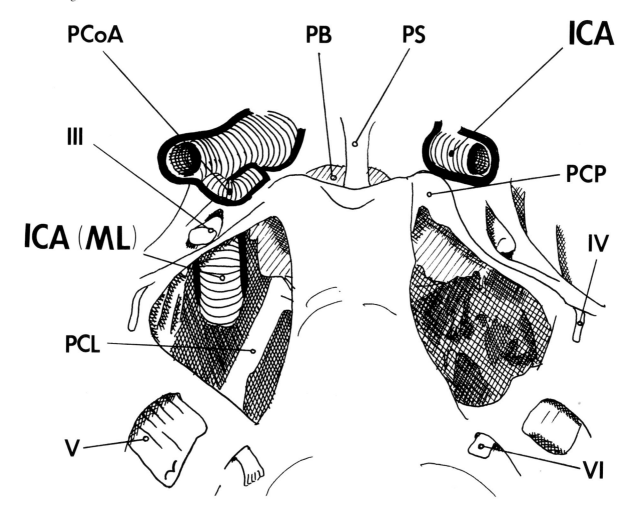

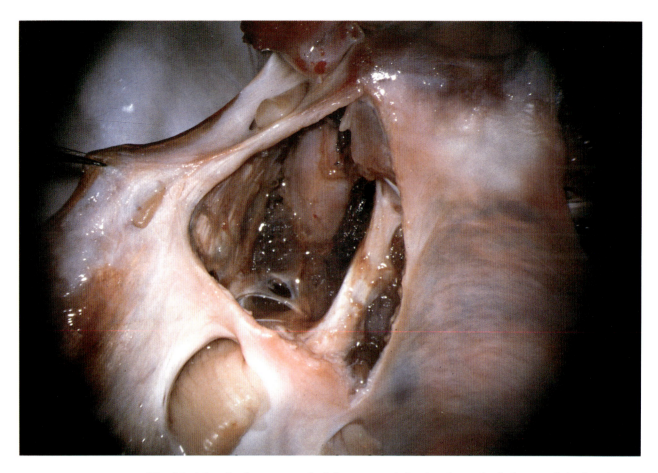

Fig. 33. After further removal of the venous injection from the inferomedial triangle, the petroclinoid ligament and its origin at the apex of the petrous bone and its insertion to the posterior aspect of the PCP are shown. The venous injection can be seen between the lateral aspect of the PCP and the medial aspect of the medial loop of the ICA. Some curvy venous trabeculae are visualized in the posterior portion of the triangle, lateral to the petroclinoid ligament and posterior to the ICA. Further removal of the venous injection from the basilar plexus, the petroclinoid ligament, the VIth nerve and the ICA, has been achieved. The network of the venous trabeculae on the lateral aspect of the petroclinoid ligament running from it to the dura is seen

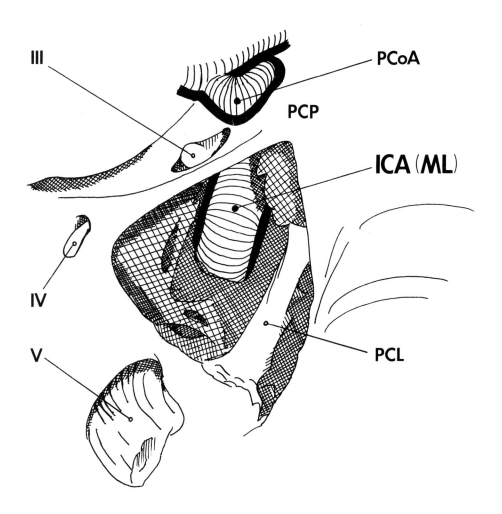

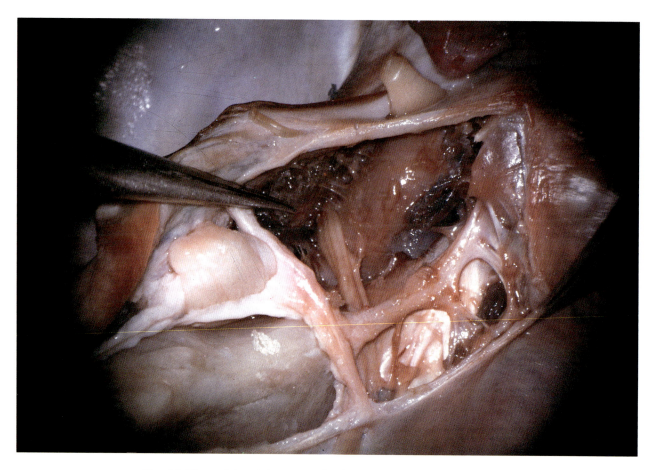

Fig. 34. The origin of the petroclinoid ligament in the apex of the petrous bone is clearly visualized. Adjacent to the tip of the apex of the petrous bone and underneath the petroclinoid ligament, the VIth nerve is shown in its entire segment from the entry point to the lateral aspect of the ICA. It can be seen that the VIth nerve is composed of five individual bundles

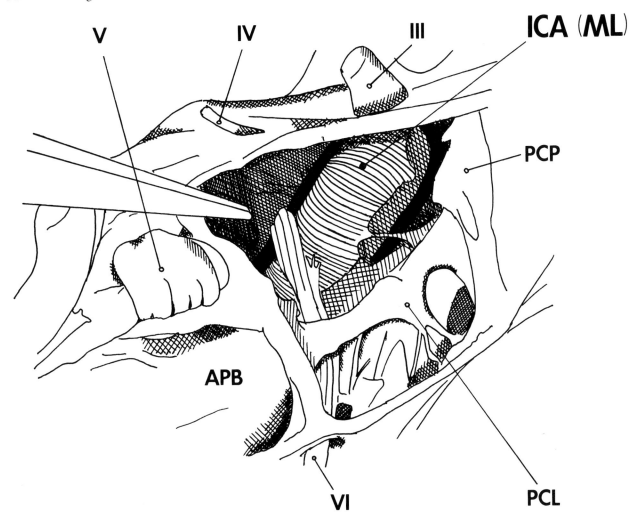

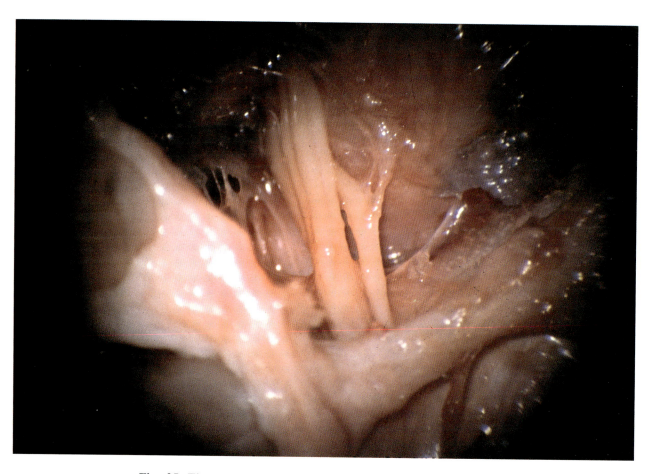

Fig. 35. The VIth nerve is shown underneath the petroclinoid ligament and under the posterior and lateral aspects of the ICA. Individual fasciculi of the VIth nerve, and sympathetic fibers running from the ICA to the VIth nerve, as well as venous trabeculae are seen

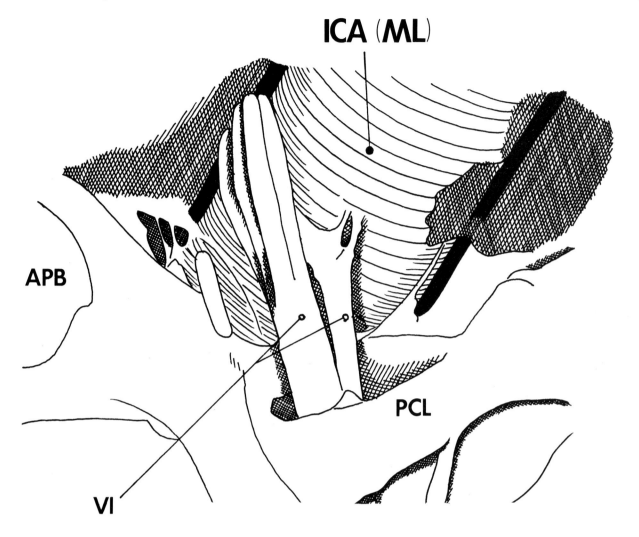

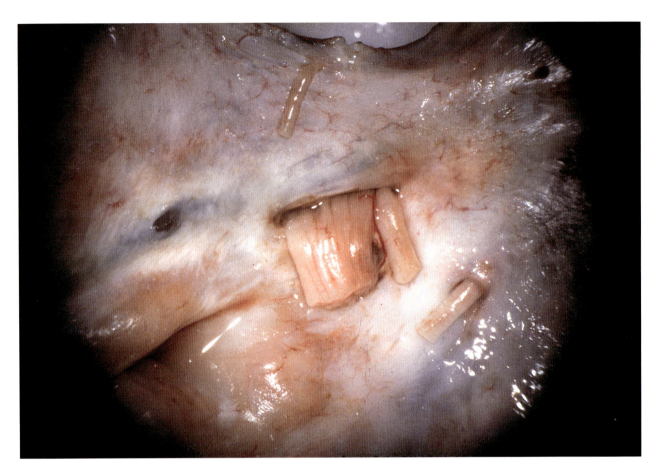

Fig. 36. The landmarks of the inferolateral (trigeminal) triangle are shown. The superomedial corner of the triangle is formed by the entry point of the IVth nerve; the inferomedial corner by the entry point of the VIth nerve; and the posterior corner by the junction of the petrous vein with the SPS. This triangle is composed of two smaller triangles: the tentorial portion above the Vth nerve and the osseous portion below the Vth nerve over the apex of the petrous bone

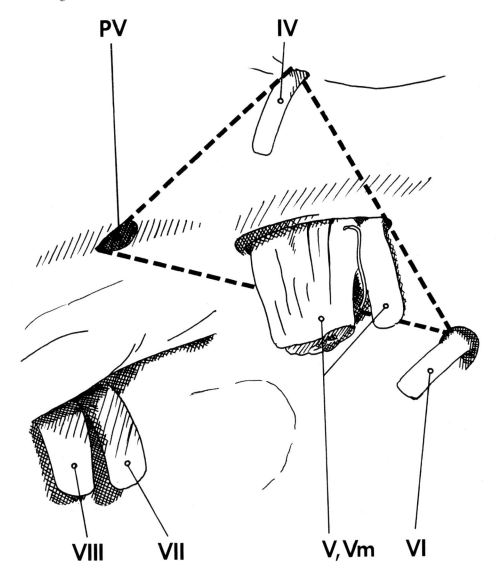

Inferolateral (trigeminal) triangle

The inferolateral triangle is defined by the dural entry point of the IVth nerve into the tentorium (superoanterior point), the dural entry point of the VIth nerve into Dorello's canal (inferomedial point), and the entry point of the petrosal vein into the SPS (lateral point). By drawing the line from the entry of the petrosal vein into the SPS to the anterior point of the exit of the Vth nerve from the posterior cranial fossa, the inferolateral triangle can be subdivided into two triangles: (a) the

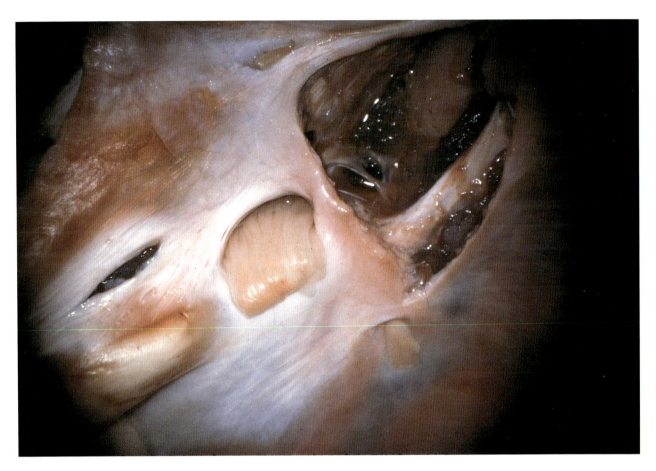

Fig. 37. The posterior corner of the inferolateral triangle, represented by the entry point of the petrous vein into the SPS, is shown. The upper and the lower corner of the inferolateral triangle represented by the entry points of the IVth and the VIth nerve respectively, are shown as well as the anterior border of the inferolateral triangle which is also the posterior border of the exposed inferomedial triangle. The Vth nerve lies in the middle of the inferolateral triangle

osseous portion formed by the dural entry point of the VIth nerve into Dorello's canal (inferomedial point), the anterior border of the Vth nerve at its entry into Meckel's cave (anterosuperior point), and the dural entry of the petrosal vein (posterosuperior point). Within this triangle, the dura overlies the posterior aspect of the petrous apex. It should be pointed out that this triangle represents the posterior fossa extension of the posteromedial (Kawase's) triangle in the middle cranial fossa (projecting through the bone of the medial petrous apex). (b) the tentorial portion, defined by the dural entry of the IVth nerve into the tentorium

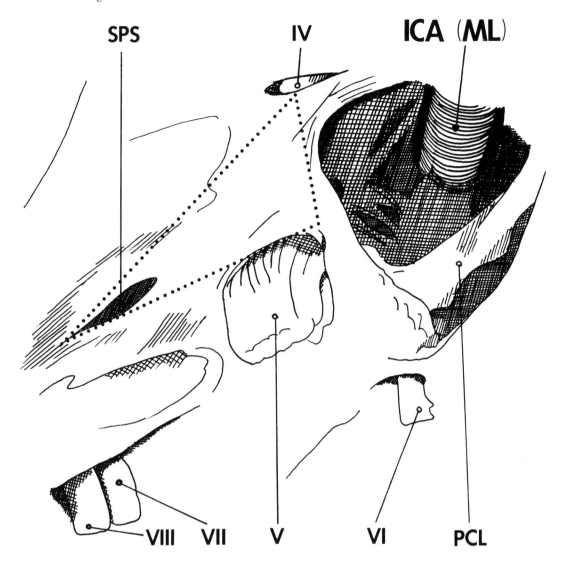

SPS   IV   ICA (ML)

VIII VII   V   VI   PCL

(superomedial point), the anterior border of the Vth nerve as it enters Meckel's cave (inferomedial point), and the dural entry point of the petrous vein (posterior point). This triangle contains a portion of the SPS and the tentorial branch of the MHT, and that portion of the tentorium cerebelli that is superoposterior to Meckel's cave.

The inferolateral triangle of the **left** CS is shown in Figs. 36–40.

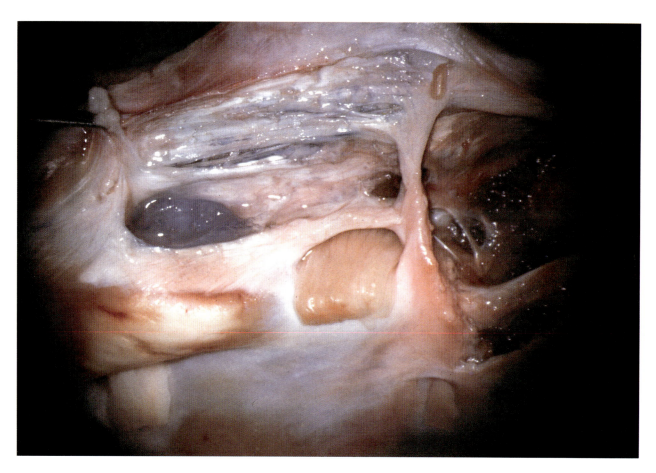

Fig. 38. The tentorial part of the inferolateral triangle is partially open. The boundary between the inferolateral and inferomedial triangles is preserved. The dura over the osseous portion of the inferolateral triangle is still in place. The SPS is partially open in the area of the entry point of the petrous vein

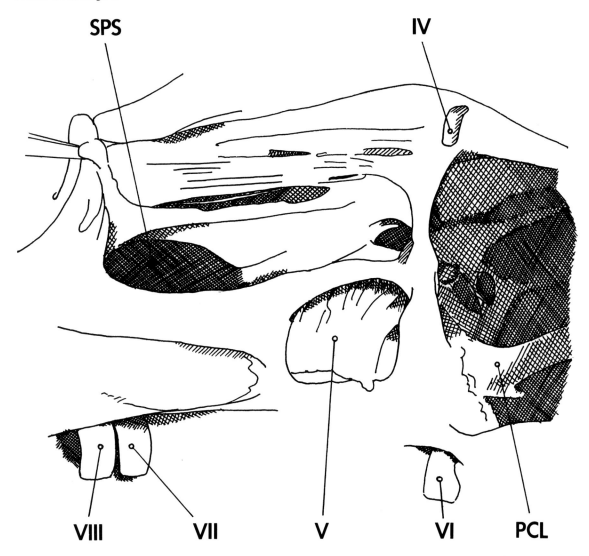

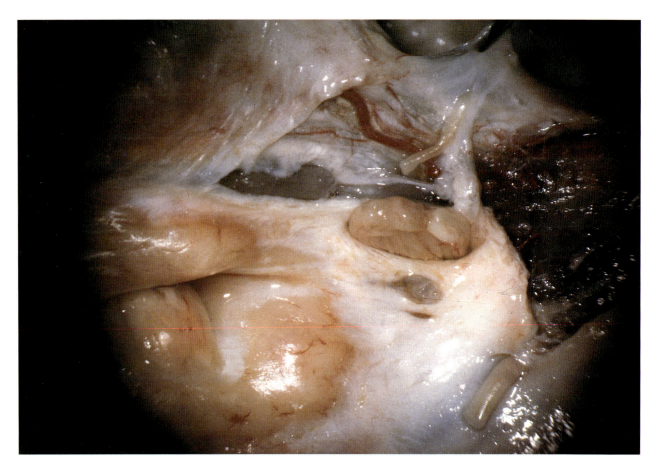

Fig. 39. The tentorial part of the inferolateral triangle has been opened and the venous injection in the SPS exposed. The venous injection is in continuity with the "venous pool" in the inferomedial triangle. The tentorial branch of the MHT is shown. The entry point of the IVth nerve representing the superomedial corner of the inferolateral triangle, and the narrow strip of the dura running from the entry point of the IVth nerve toward the anterior corner of the entry point of the Vth nerve representing the anterior border of the tentorial portion of the inferolateral triangle, are seen

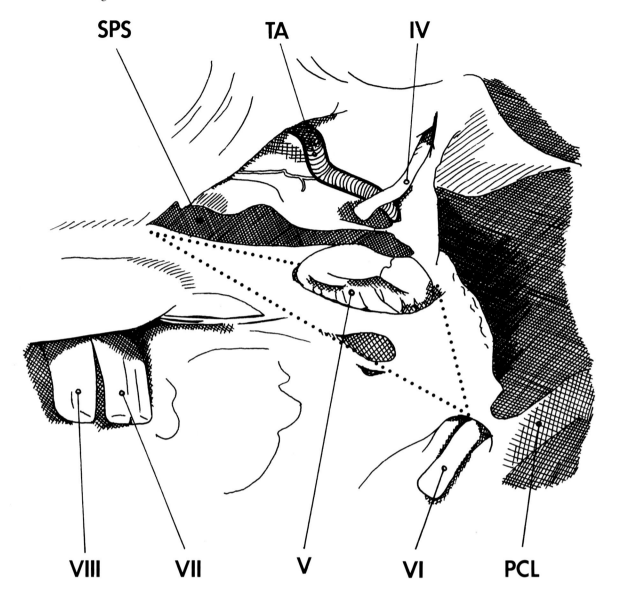

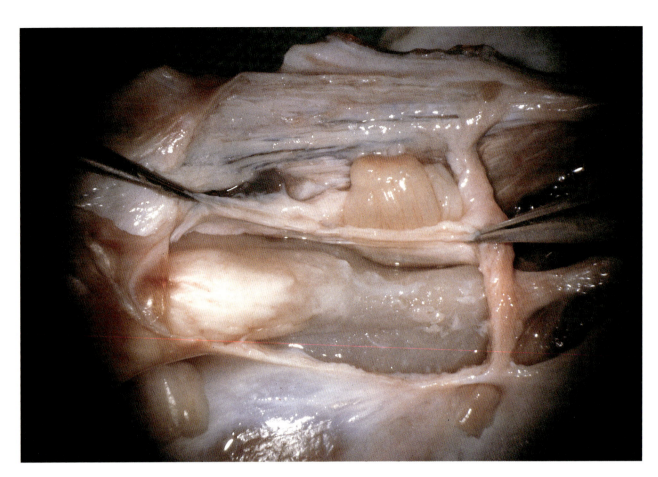

Fig. 40. The dura over the apex of the petrous bone is excised and the osseous portion of the inferolateral triangle is exposed. The Vth nerve is covered on its under aspect toward the apex of the petrous bone with the dural layer. From the entry point of the IVth nerve to the entry point of the VIth nerve, a narrow strip of the dura is preserved representing the boundary between the inferolateral and inferomedial triangles. The petroclinoid ligament originates at the very tip of the apex of petrous bone. The inner auditory canal is very close to the dorsolateral aspect of the apex of the petrous bone which represents the osseous portion of the inferolateral triangle. At operation, when drilling the apex of the petrous bone from the middle fossa toward the posterior fossa dorsal to the Vth nerve, the direction of the drilling should be anteromedial

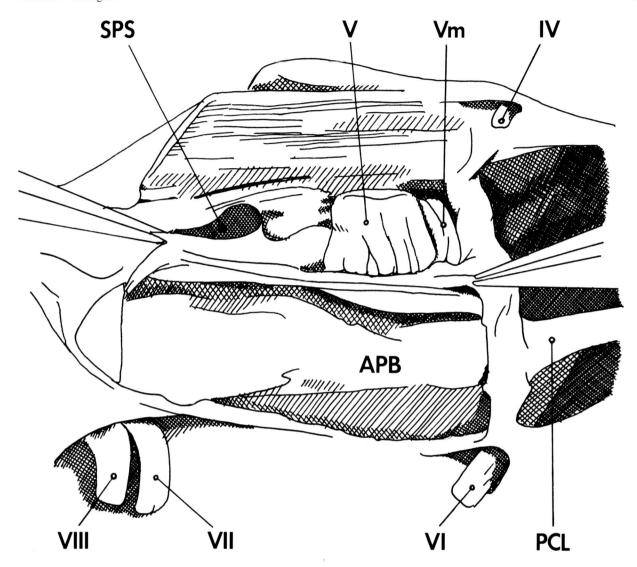

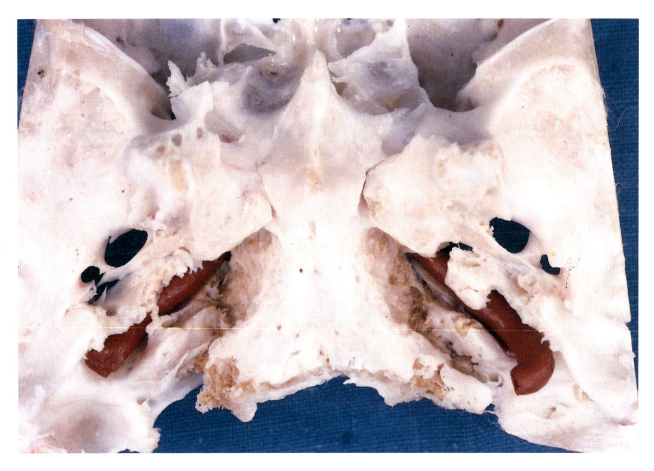

Fig. 41. The inferior aspect of the bony structures of the skull base shows the two ICAs entering the respective carotid canals into the petrous bone. The thin bone of the carotid canal under both ICAs is removed. Immediately after entering the bony canal in the petrous bone, the ICA turns from its vertical course in an anteromedial direction and runs in an almost horizontal plane to the foramen lacerum. The turn which the ICA makes in the carotid canal in the petrous bone is called the posterior loop

1.3 Relation of the internal carotid artery to the surgical triangles and bony sinuses

At the skull base the ICA extends from the inferoposterolateral corner toward the superoanteromedial corner. In its course at the skull base it forms four loops: the posterior, lateral, medial, and anterior loop. Each loop lies in a different plane suggesting that the artery spins around its longitudinal axis as does the blood flow

FO   FS

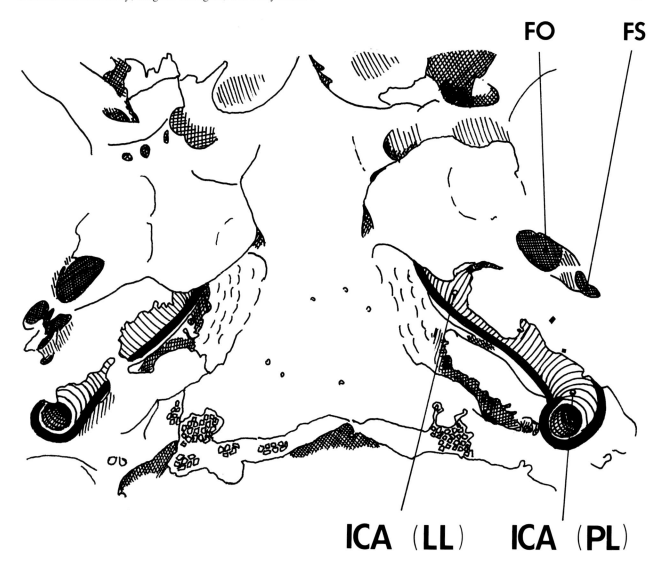

ICA (LL)   ICA (PL)

in it. The phenomenon of blood spin is believed to have some bearing on blood temperature.

Aneurysms of the ICA in the carotid canal of the petrous bone and in the segment underneath the fibrous layer proximal to the lateral ring, occur only occasionally and are less dangerous. Conversely, tumorous lesions can easily grow along the ICA into the canal, an indication for the exposure of the ICA in the petrous bone in order to delineate the extent of the tumor, especially when the tumor is benign and when complete resection is attempted.

Most traumatic aneuryms of the ICA in the CS are located in the segment of the

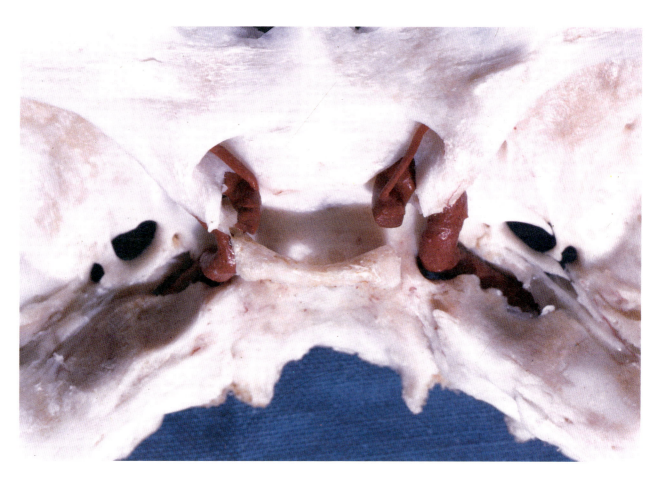

Fig. 42. At the foramen lacerum the ICA turns upward and medially forming the lateral loop. From the foramen lacerum, the ICA runs toward the PCP where it turns forward, forming the medial loop adjacent to the PCP. From the PCP, the ICA runs horizontally, inferolateral to the ACP, making a U-turn around it, thus forming the anterior loop

ICA between the proximal and distal dural rings and project anteromedially into the sphenoid sinus.

The entire course of the ICA at the skull base on the **left** side is presented in Figs. 41–55.

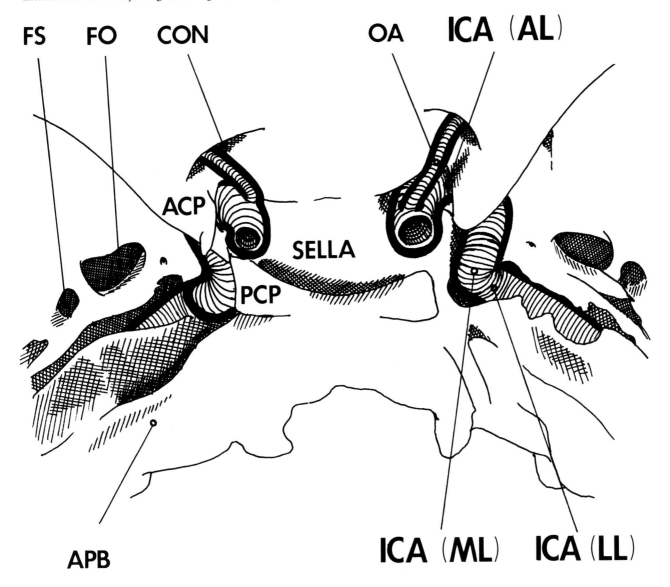

FS FO CON

OA ICA (AL)

ACP

SELLA

PCP

APB

ICA (ML) ICA (LL)

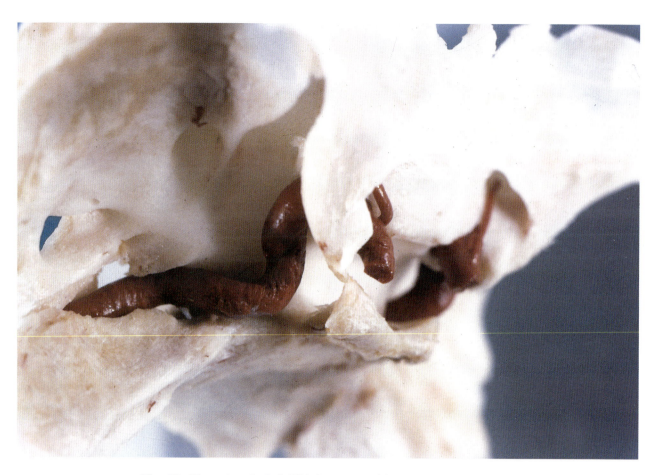

Fig. 43. Observing the left ICA from a semi-lateral direction, the entire course of the ICA at the skull base can be represented by two consecutive S-segments so that the second S-segment is the direct continuation of the first one. The first S-segments of the ICA represents the posterior and lateral loops of the artery whereas the second S-segment represents its medial and anterior loops. The junction of the two S-segments is level with the tip of the apex of the petrous bone and represents the border between the covered and free segments of the ICA at the skull base

FO   FLa   FR   SOF   ICA (AL)   OA   CON

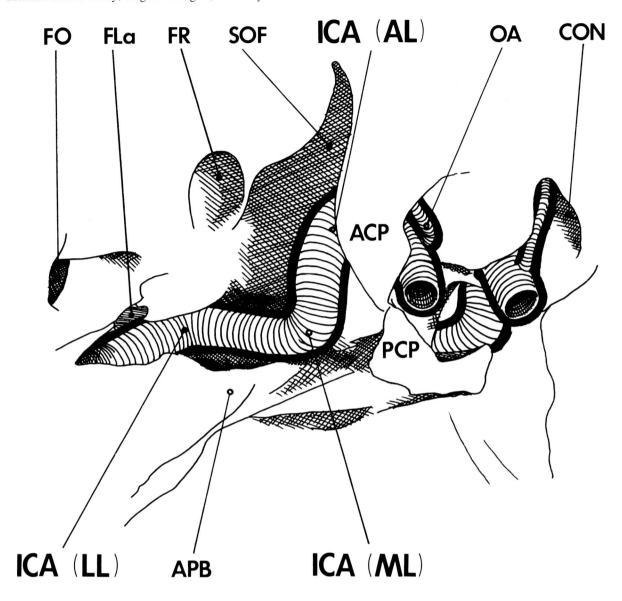

ACP

PCP

ICA (LL)   APB   ICA (ML)

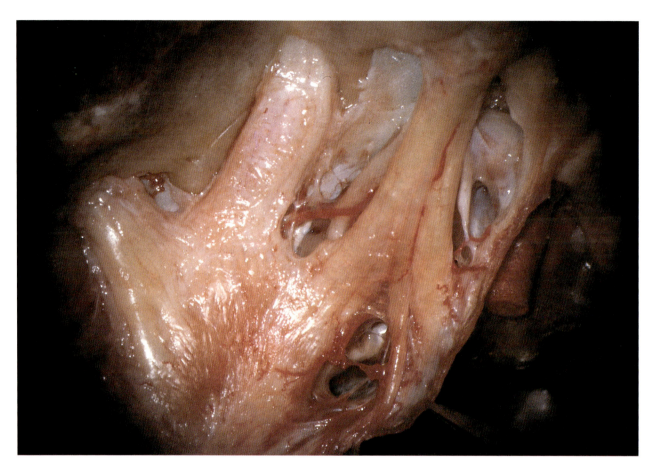

Fig. 44. The anterior loop of the ICA is seen through the anteromedial triangle whereas the medial loop of the ICA is seen through Parkinson's triangle. Through the anterolateral triangle, a small portion of the ICA at its exit from the petrous bone can be seen underneath the fibrous bridge overlying the ICA and forming the so-called lateral rings of the ICA. Through the anterolateral triangle a large branch of the ILT and the VIth nerve are seen. The lateral ring of the ICA represents the junction of the two S-segments of the ICA at the skull base: the first S-segment, consisting of the posterior and lateral loops of the ICA, is covered by the fibrous membrane under the GG and by bone in the carotid canal of the petrous bone whereas the second intracavernous S-segment, consisting of the medial and anterior loops, is free

V3   V2   VI   V1   PR   MM   DR   OA

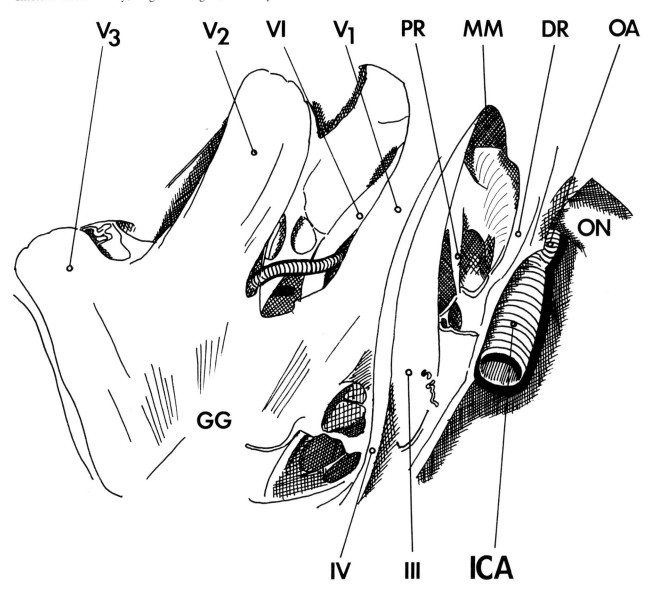

ON

IV   III   ICA

GG

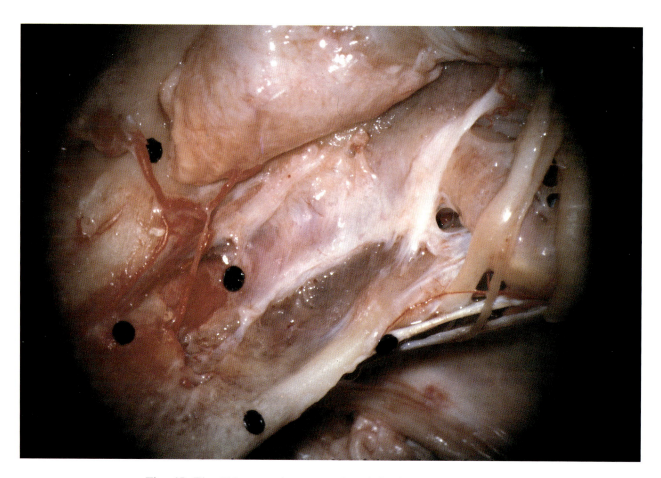

Fig. 45. The Vth nerve is retracted and the lateral ring around the ICA is shown. The lateral loop of the ICA under the Vth nerve and medial to Meckel's cave is covered by a fibrous membrane. The sympathetic nerves running along the ICA under the fibrous covering turn away at the exit of the ICA from the lateral ring to join the VIth nerve. Posterior to the Vth nerve the ICA in the carotid canal is partially unroofed. The posterolateral and posteromedial triangles are marked with black dots at their corners

MMA   LR   SNN

GG

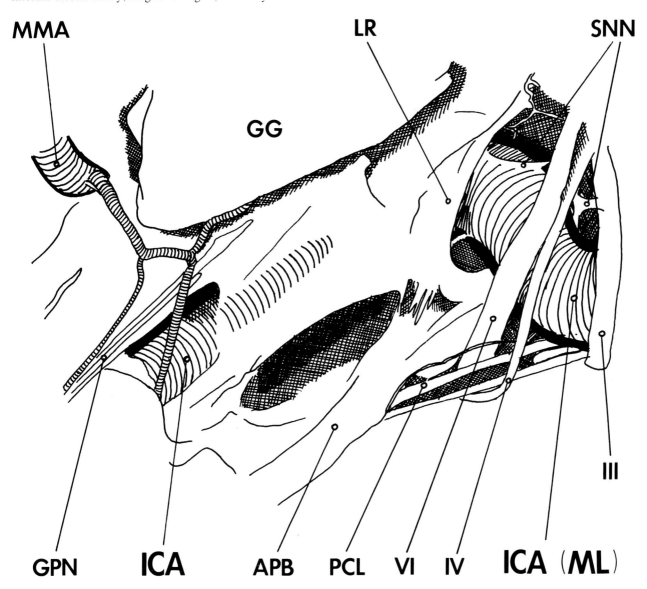

III

GPN   **ICA**   APB   PCL   VI   IV   **ICA (ML)**

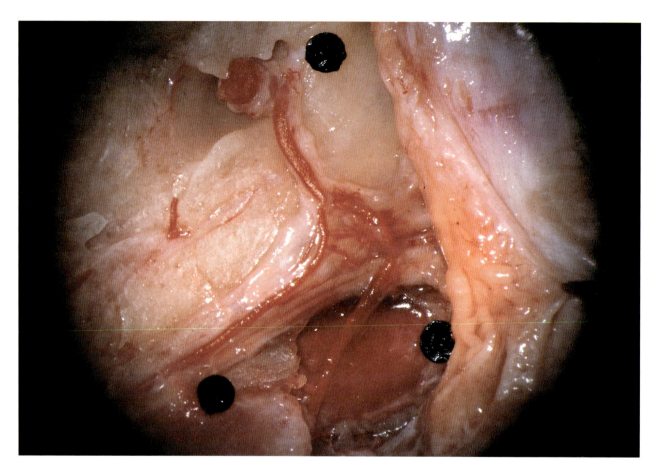

Fig. 46. The posterolateral triangle and the middle meningeal artery are indicated. The middle meningeal artery and its branches accompanying the greater petrosal nerve are seen. The distal segment of the posterior loop of the ICA is shown running forward to the foramen lacerum. The greater petrosal nerve courses lateral to and above the ICA toward the foramen lacerum. In all cases in which it is planned to explore the whole CS during surgery, the presented segment of the ICA should be exposed. At this stage the ICA provides the surgeon with very valuable information about its position under the Vth nerve. In some cases, the ICA may run more laterally toward the foramen lacerum, in others, more medially

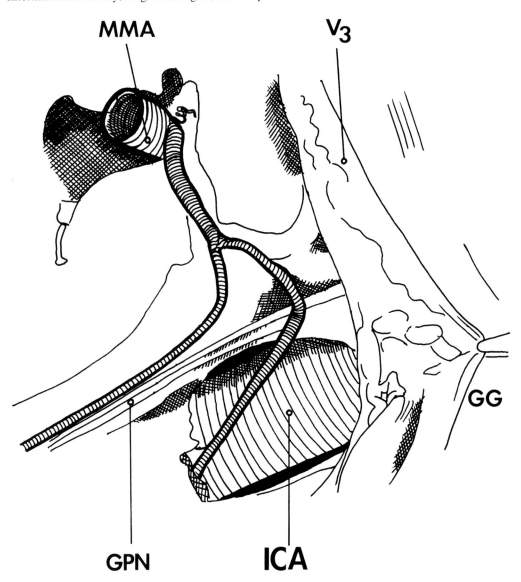

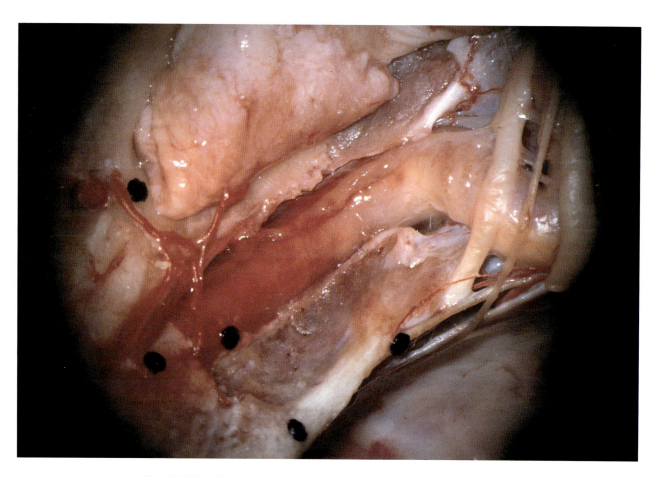

Fig. 47. The fibrous membrane above the lateral loop of the ICA with its lateral ring is wide open. Part of the ICA is exposed in the carotid canal. The large sympathetic fibers accompanying the ICA and joining the VIth nerve are visualized. This figure, as well as Fig. 45, offers a fairly reasonable explanation as to why the most frequent site of aneurysms is between the lateral and proximal rings on the intracavernous ICA

MMA   SN   ICA (LL)   III

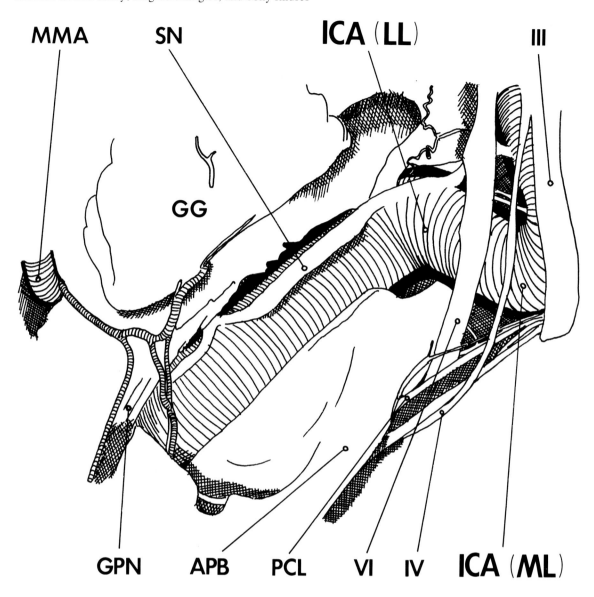

GG

GPN   APB   PCL   VI   IV   ICA (ML)

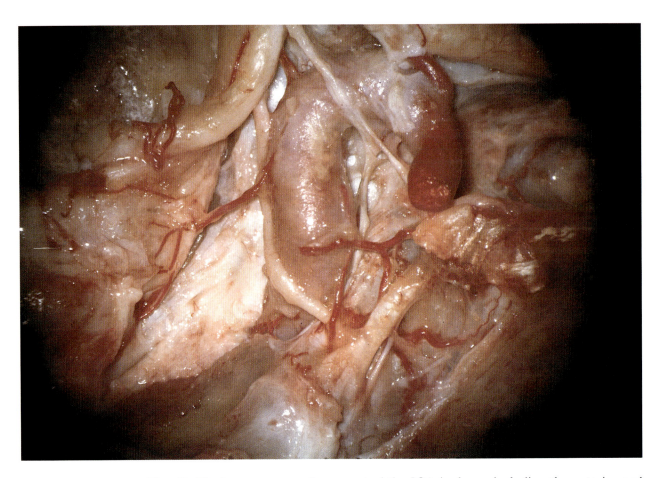

Fig. 48. The intracavernous S-segment of the ICA is shown including the anterior and medial loops of the ICA. It is also evident that the anterior and medial loops are in the horizontal and in the sagittal plane, respectively. All the nerves running in the lateral wall of the CS have been elevated but the VIth nerve has been left in place. In the CS the VIth nerve runs inferior and lateral to the MHT and the ILT. The proximal and distal dural rings of the anterior loop of the ICA are shown. The proximal ring is fixed to the PCP. The extracavernous and intracavernous portions of the anterior loop are shown

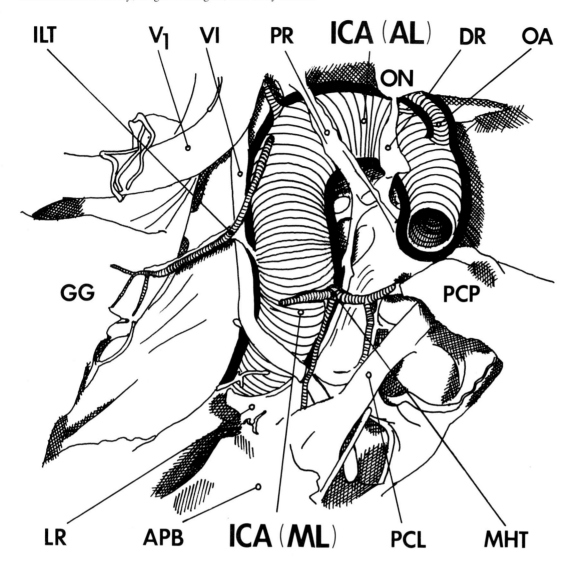

ILT V₁ VI PR **ICA (AL)** DR OA

ON

GG

PCP

LR APB **ICA (ML)** PCL MHT

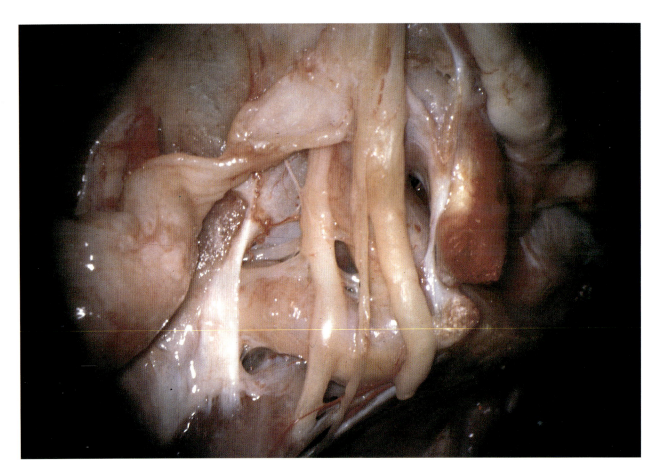

Fig. 49. The intracavernous segment of the ICA is shown from its exit from the lateral ring to the distal dural rings. From the ICA the sympathetic fibers run to the VIth nerve joining it at different sites. Thus the VIth nerve is actually attached to the ICA in the CS. The IIIrd and the IVth nerves, running almost parallel to the horizontal segment of the ICA, are not fixed to the artery but are, like V1, located in the lateral wall of the CS

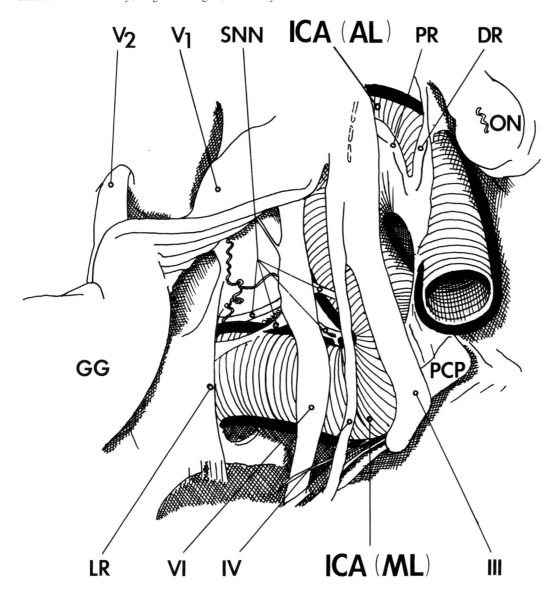

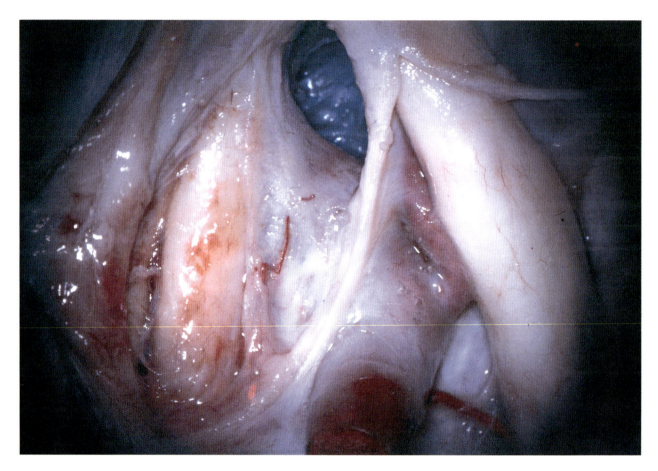

Fig. 50. In the anteromedial triangle the anterior loop of the ICA is fixed with the proximal and distal dural rings to the bone for a length equal to almost three quarters of its circumference. The fibrous proximal ring of the ICA, firmly attached to the anteroinferior surface of the ACP and to the ICA, prevents mobility of the artery in its course from the proximal to the distal dural ring. This is of paramount importance in cases of bone fracture at the ICA, which may result in traumatic aneurysm

PR MM DR OA

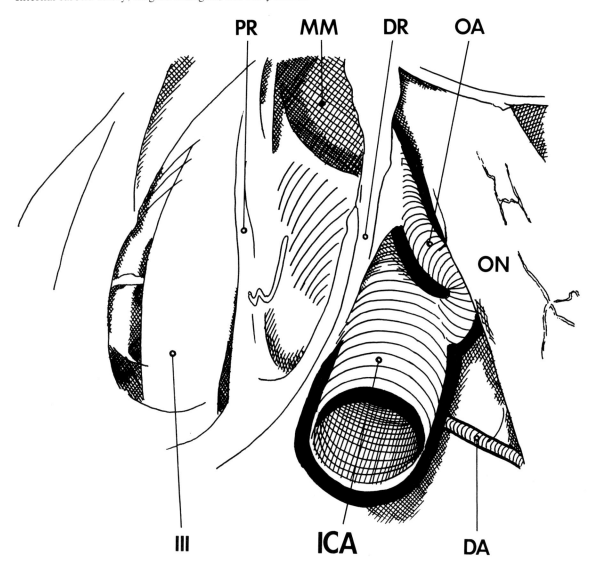

III ICA DA

ON

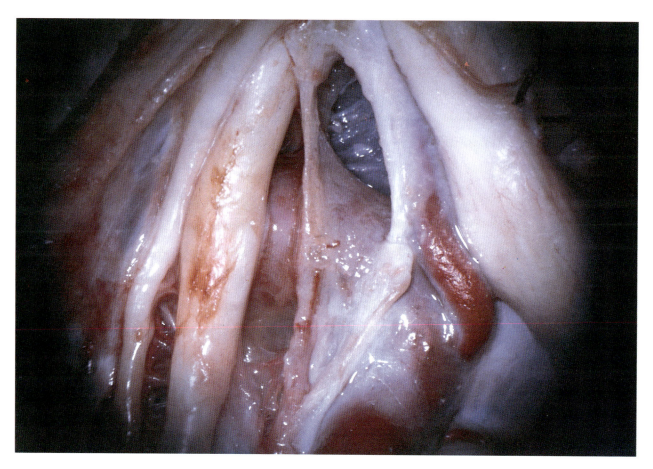

Fig. 51. The proximal ring fixed to the distal dural ring and to the PCP and along the lateral aspect of the ACP and anteriorly to the dura covering the SOF, is firm and holds the anterior loop of the ICA in place. The proximal ring forms the border of the CS and also the border of intracavernous aneurysms: proximal to the proximal ring aneurysms occur frequently, whereas distal to it they are unusual, except when they are traumatic

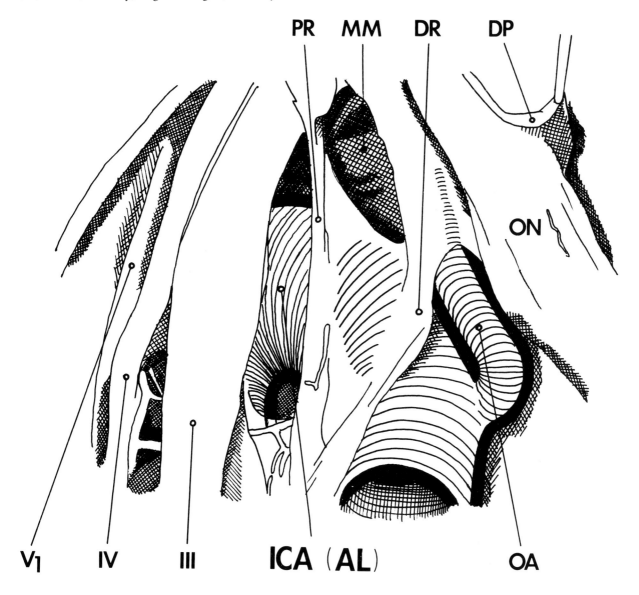

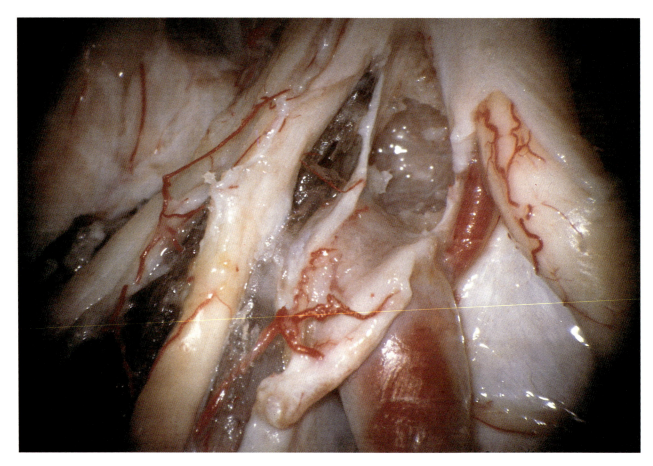

Fig. 52. The anterior loop of the ICA is somewhat protected in the segment between the proximal and distal dural rings. Most surgical procedures in the CS require the removal of the ACP and complete exposure of the anterior loop of the ICA. It is very important to be familiar with the extreme vulnerability of the thin bony wall of the sphenoid sinus on the medial and anterior aspects of the anterior loop of the ICA. If this wall is damaged and the mucous membrane perforated, a CSF leak will result unless the wall is repaired with muscle and fibrin glue

V₁ ICA (AL) MM ON

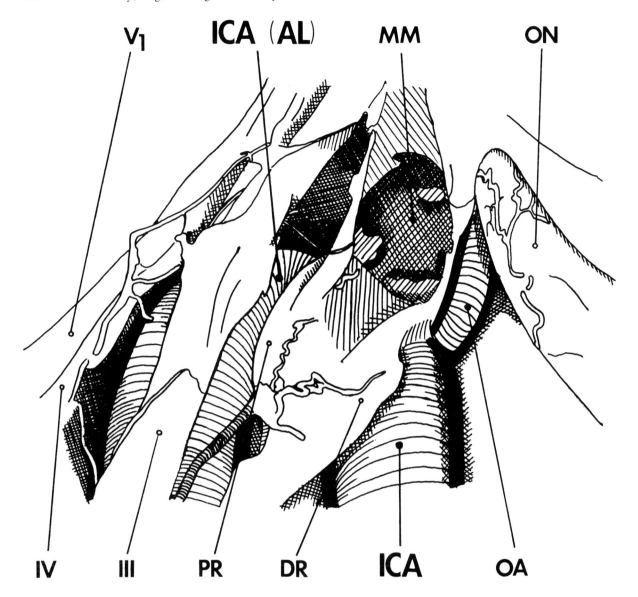

IV III PR DR ICA OA

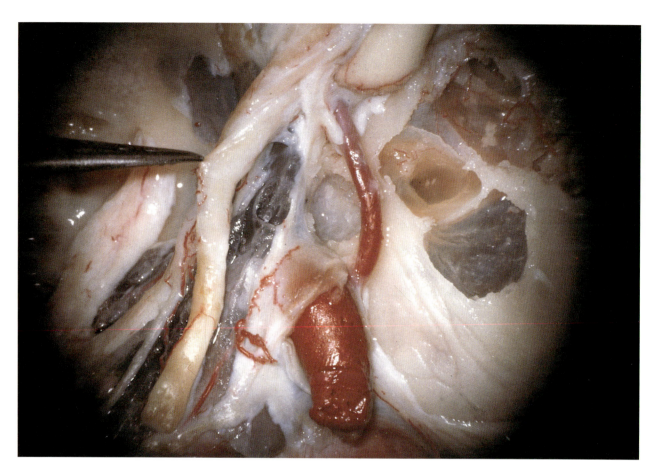

Fig. 53. The dura propria has been cut along the longitudinal axis of the ON and the ON has been elevated, so that the ophthalmic artery can be seen. At the corner between the ICA and the ophthalmic artery, the wall of the ethmoid sinus has been damaged. The venous injection under the IIIrd, IVth, VIth, and V1 nerves can be seen. The proximal ring is on the anteromedial border of the CS

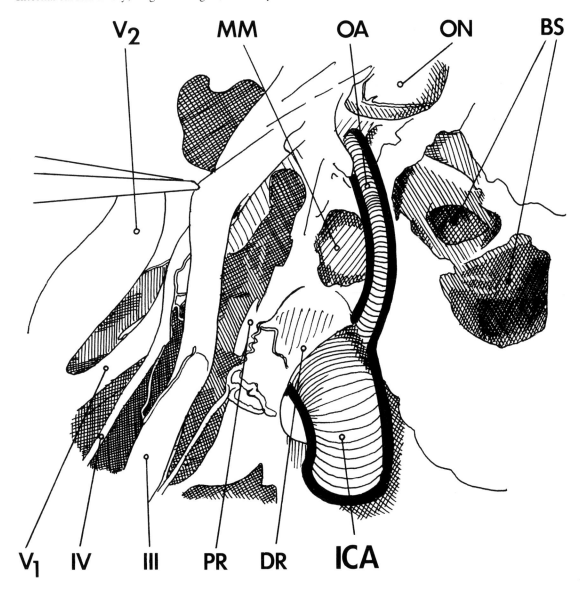

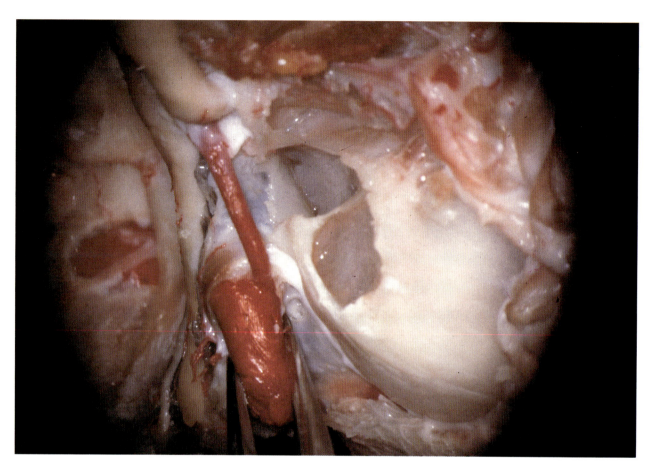

Fig. 54. The ON has been elevated. The ophthalmic artery can be visualized. On further rotation of the specimen to the left, the very thin bony wall of the sphenoid sinus, to which the segment of the anterior loop of the ICA between the proximal and distal rings is attached, can be seen. Medial to the intradural portion of the ICA a part of the pituitary body is seen. Since the thickness of the sphenoid sinus wall is variable, opening of the innermost wall too far laterally during transsphenoidal surgery of the sellar lesion may result in injury to the ICA and false aneurysm. Note that the anterior loop of the ICA is practically perpendicular to the posterior loop of the ICA

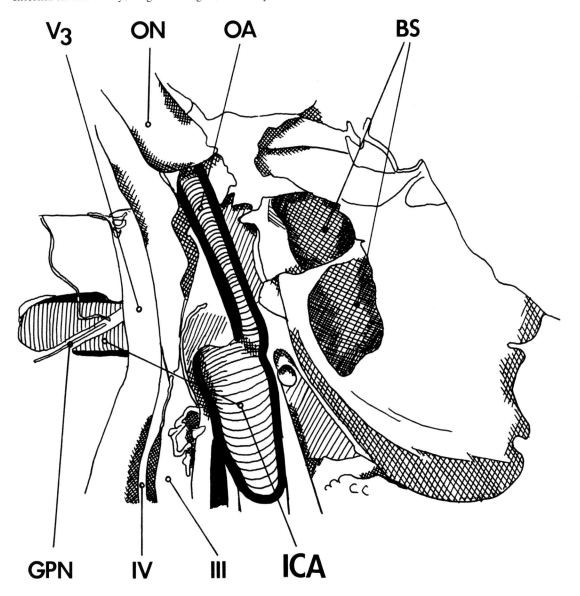

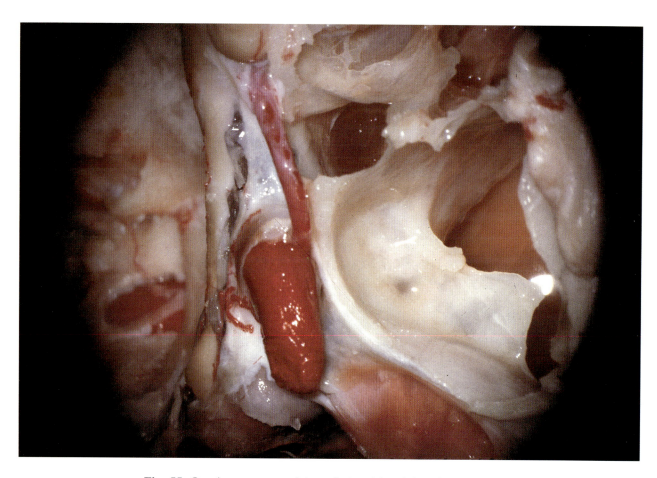

Fig. 55. One is not aware of the relationship of the ICA to the bony sinuses and the sella when working only from the intracranial side or only through the sphenoid sinus. Only by visualizing the ICA and the bony sinuses simultaneously from above one realises that the bony sinuses may be entered accidentally from the intracranial direction, with a resultant CSF leak, or the ICA may be injured from the opposite side with a resultant traumatic ICA aneurysm

V3   OA   BS

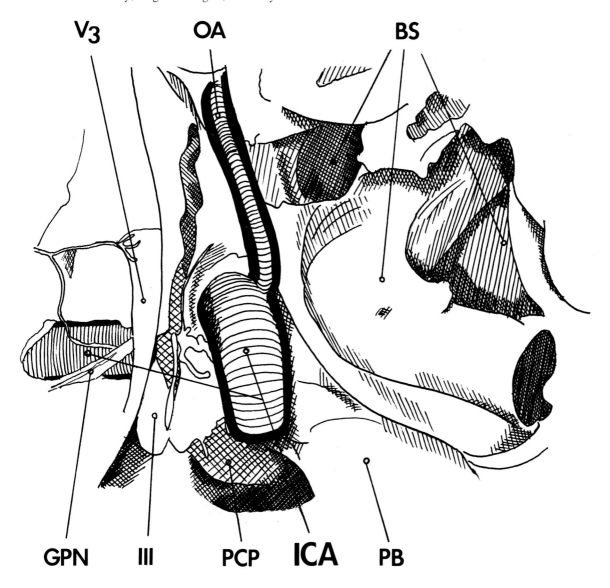

GPN   III   PCP   **ICA**   PB

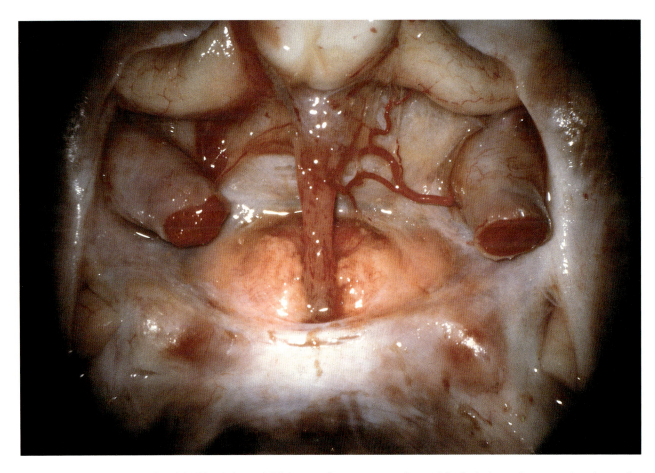

Fig. 56. The injected ICAs can be seen together with their branches running from the medial aspect of the ICA on either side toward the pituitary stalk, optic chiasm, and optic nerves. The intradural segment of the ICA from the ACP to the PCP is seen running parallel to the horizontal segment of the ICA in the CS

1.4 Relation of the cavernous sinus to the sella

The sella with the pituitary body is in the central position and has for its lateral borders the left and right CSs. Both CSs communicate with each other through the intercavernous sinuses inside the sella, on its floor, and its anterior and posterior walls. The arterial supply of the capsule of the pituitary body is provided by branches from the ICA in the CS whereas the supply of the pituitary stalk is provided by branches from the ICA shortly after its entry into the intradural space.

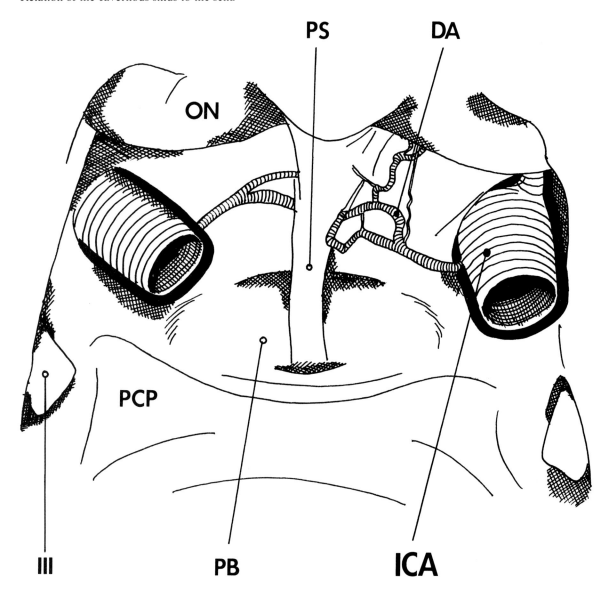

The hormones of the pituitary body are released into the venous blood around it. Tumors of the CS may grow into the sella and may compress the pituitary body, causing changes in its endocrine functions. Conversely, a tumor of the pituitary body may easily compress or invade the parasellar space and cause symptoms of involvement of the IIIrd, IVth, Vth, and VIth nerves.

The relation of the CS to the sella is presented in Figs. 56–61.

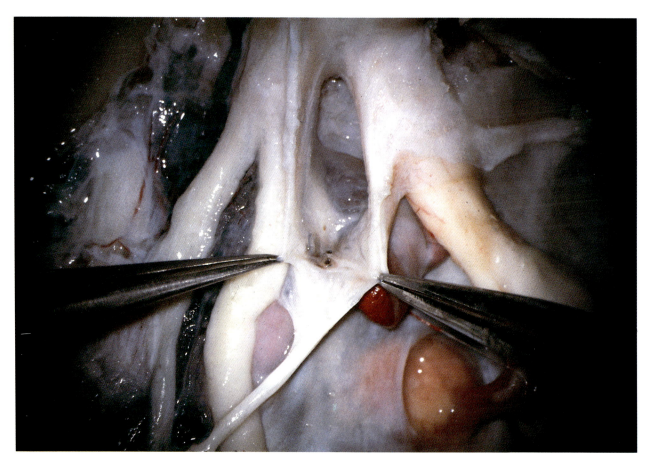

Fig. 57. After removal of the tip of the left ACP, the venous injection is seen in the area of the anteromedial triangle. This means that the tip of the ACP can also be located in the CS and medial to the horizontal segment of the ICA. In surgery, during removal of the ACP, venous bleeding from the CS may be triggered only when the last piece of the tip of the ACP is removed. In some cases, the ACP is very long and projects far posteriorly, or may be in continuity with the PCP. Frequently a long ACP projects far medially into the sella. In this specimen, abundant venous injection can also be seen medial to the ICA toward the pituitary body. The transparent dura shows blue in the area of the oculomotor triangle

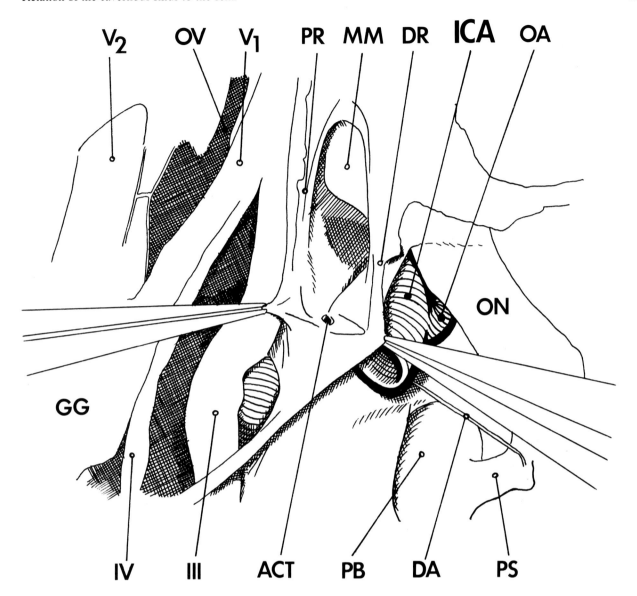

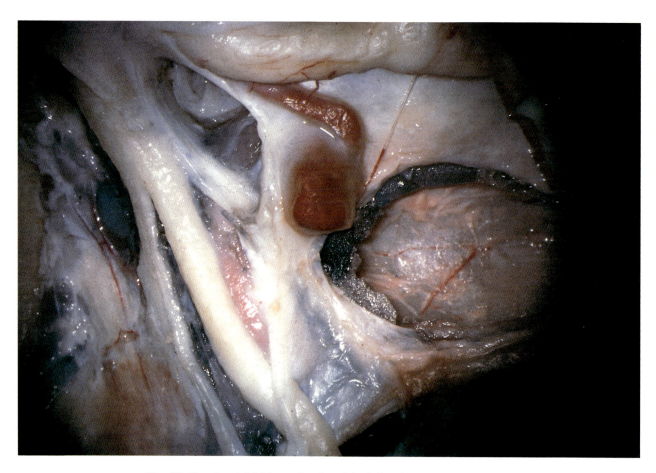

Fig. 58. The dural fold from the tip of the left PCP to the tip of the removed ACP represents the medial border of the oculomotor trigone and is also the direct continuation of the proximal ring around the ICA. The distal dural ring of the ICA continues toward the entry point of the IIIrd nerve fixing, firstly, the proximal ring around the ICA and, secondly, the dural fold running from the PCP to the ACP. The pituitary body has been removed and venous injection can be seen at the bottom of the sella and on its anterior and dorsal walls. The intercavernous sinus at the bottom of the sella is covered with a thin membrane displaying a network of thin arterial branches originating in the two ICAs in the CSs

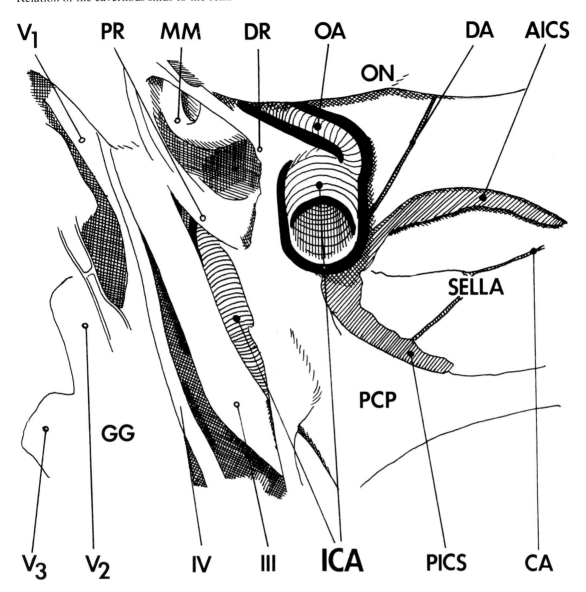

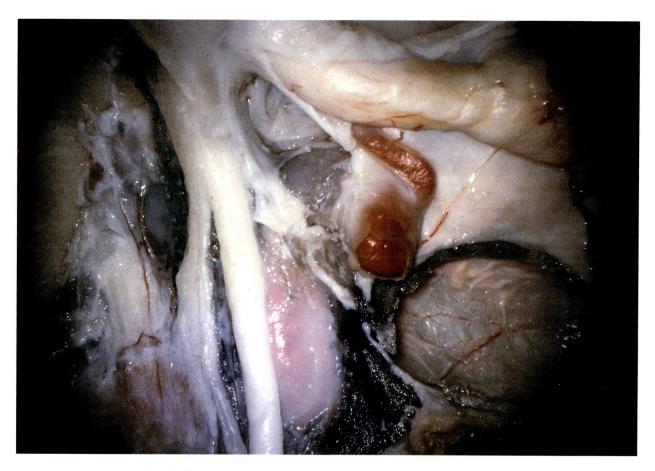

Fig. 59. Further resection of the dura in the area of the oculomotor triangle together with the dural fold running from the left PCP to the two dural rings and the ACP reveals that the connection continues into the depth forming the gentle fibrous curtain between the sella and the CS. The rich venous injection is also seen medial to the horizontal segment of the ICA and in continuation with the intercavernous sinuses

V2 V1 PR MM DR OA DA ON

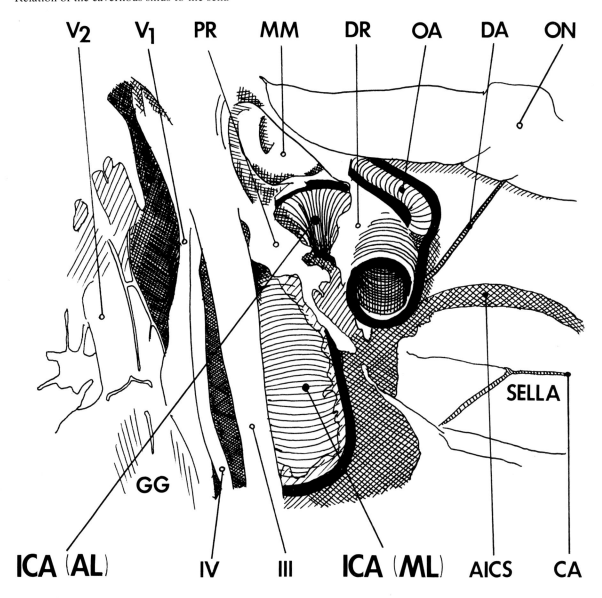

ICA (AL) IV III ICA (ML) AICS CA

GG

SELLA

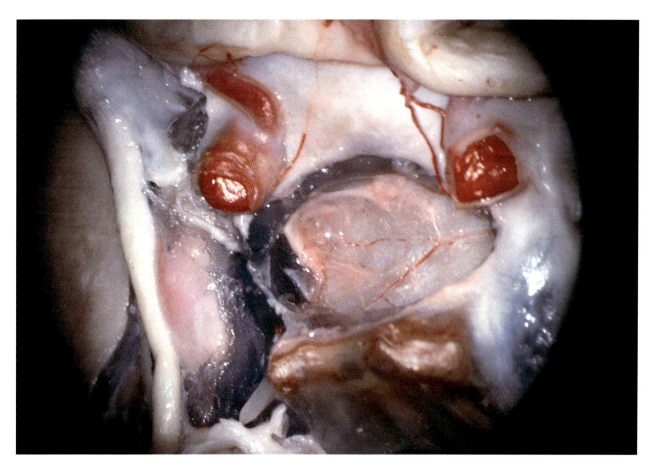

Fig. 60. Further excision of the capsule of the pituitary body at the bottom of the sella shows an even more abundant venous injection in the sella medial to the ICA and lateral to the pituitary body. In the thin curtain dividing the sella from the parasellar space, a tiny window is shown through which the intercavernous sinus in continuity with the CS on the left side is seen. The arterial injection visualizes the delicate branches in the capsule of the pituitary body at the bottom of the sella. On the right side of the sella, at the level of the PCP, blue color is seen through the transparent dura. The large intercavernous sinuses situated around the pituitary body inside the sella offer ample space for tumor growth from the sella to the parasellar region or in the opposite direction

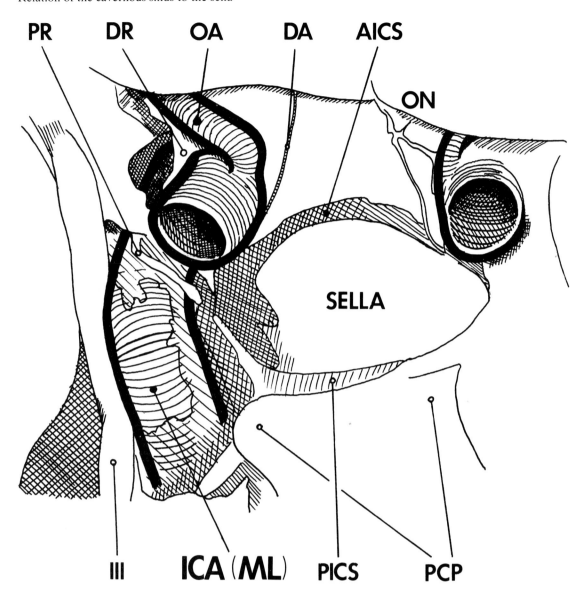

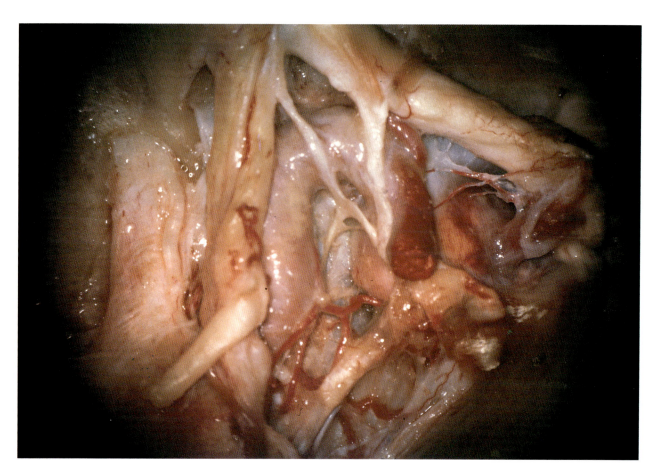

Fig. 61. The anterior and medial loops of the left ICA are shown. The proximal and distal dural rings with their attachment to the PCP and to the floor of the sella are presented. Arising from the medial loop of the ICA, the MHT with its branches can be seen. The petroclinoid ligament and the VIth nerve running under its lateral portion from Dorello's canal posterior to the lateral side of the ICA are shown. The IIIrd, IVth, and V1 nerves run on the lateral aspect of the horizontal segment of the ICA. On the medial aspect of the anteromedial triangle, the ON covered by dura propria and the ophthalmic artery located intrathecally are visible. The arteries running from the inferomedial aspect of the intradural segment of the ICA to the ON, the optic chiasm, the pituitary stalk, and the pituitary body are shown. It can be seen that the best approach to the sella and the pituitary body is through the anteromedial triangle and from the lateral aspect of the intradural ICA. After removal of the ACP epidurally and the opening of the anteromedial triangle, the corridor through the U-space of the anterior loop of the ICA offers an ideal approach to the bottom of the sella. This approach to intrasellar tumors is the alternative to transsphenoidal surgery. On the other hand, tumors spreading beyond the sellar boundaries into the CS can be radically resected because the transcavernous approach offers a sufficiently good view of all the structures in and around the sella

V₂   V₁   IV   PR   **ICA (AL)**   DR   OA   ON   DA

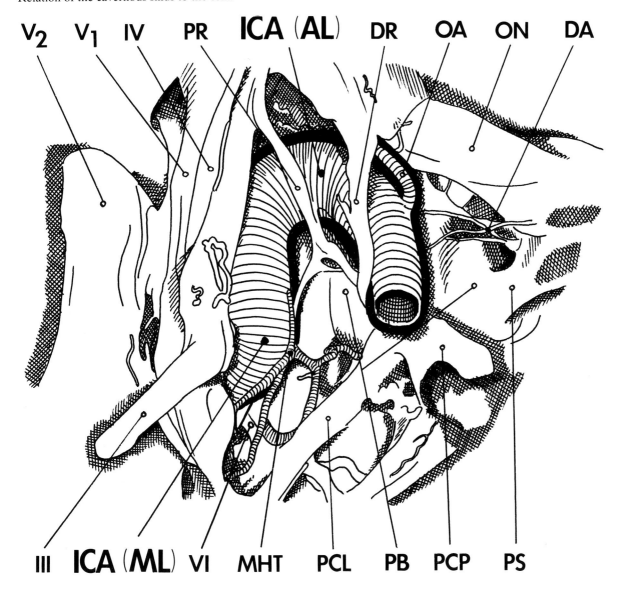

III   **ICA (ML)**   VI   MHT   PCL   PB   PCP   PS

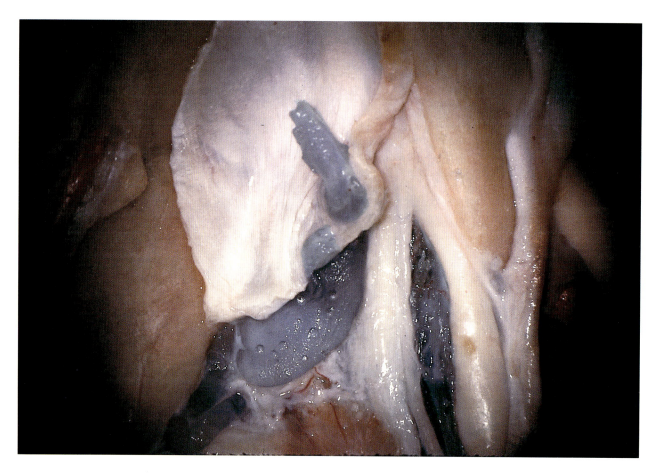

Fig. 62. The venous injection of the left CS shows a large brain surface draining vein entering the lateral wall of the CS and forming a pool of "venous blood" between the two layers of the lateral wall of the CS

1.5 Venous system of the cavernous sinuses

The main veins supplying the CSs on each side are the superior and inferior ophthalmic veins, the sphenoparietal sinus, and rather variable veins draining the brain. Sometimes these veins are very large and the drainage from the brain into the CS considerable. In other cases this drainage is minimal or almost non-existent. The main route for the blood flow from the CSs is through the paired superior and inferior petrous sinuses. Considerable blood from the CSs is also

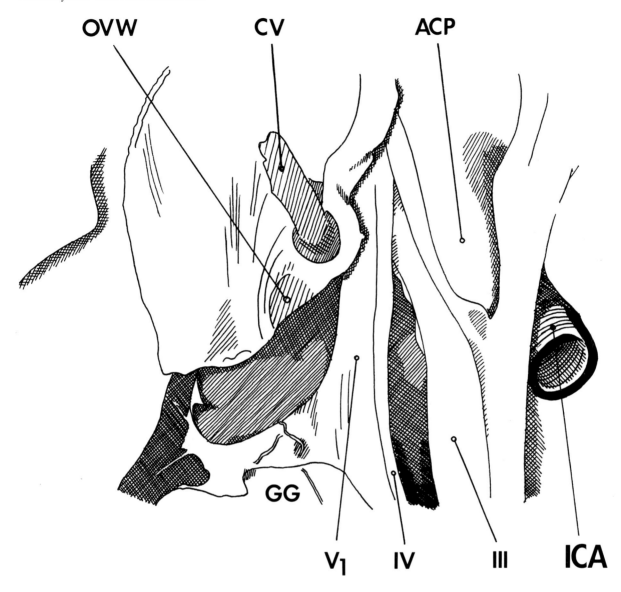

OVW **CV** **ACP**

GG

V₁ **IV** **III** **ICA**

drained via other foramina at the skull base. The CS filled with either a large or giant aneurysm or a tumor, is almost without venous blood on that side. When the CS is only partially blocked by the lesion, the main venous stream is displaced to one or to the other corner of the CS. In view of the above, it is much easier to control venous bleeding in a CS with a lesion than it is in a CS with no lesion. Gradual occlusion of the major part of a CS by a tumor and additional occlusion of

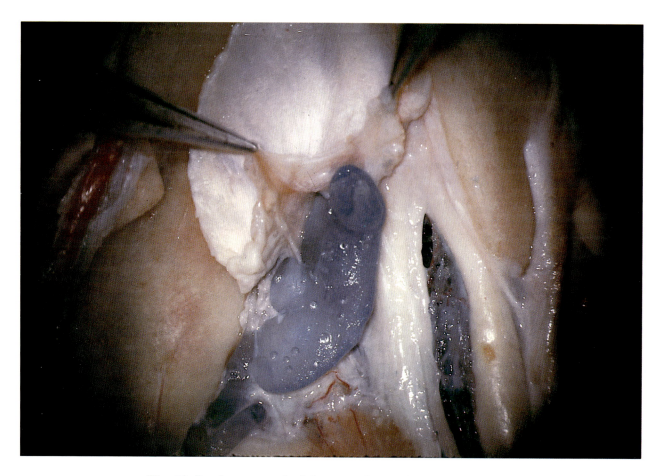

Fig. 63. Further removal of the outer layer of the lateral wall of the CS from the vein entering the CS shows a huge collection of »venous blood« between the two layers of the lateral wall of the CS. The venous injection is also seen in the paramedial triangle and laterally in the lateral triangle

the remaining functioning part of the CS during surgery does not result in ipsilateral exophthalmos. In acute infection or in some cases of pseudotumor, however, acute and complete occlusion of the CS will result in exophthalmos.

The venous system of the **left** CS is shown in Figs. 62–65.

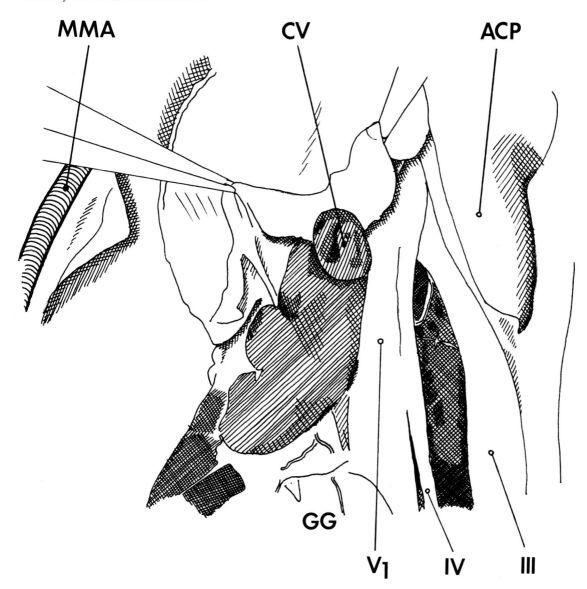

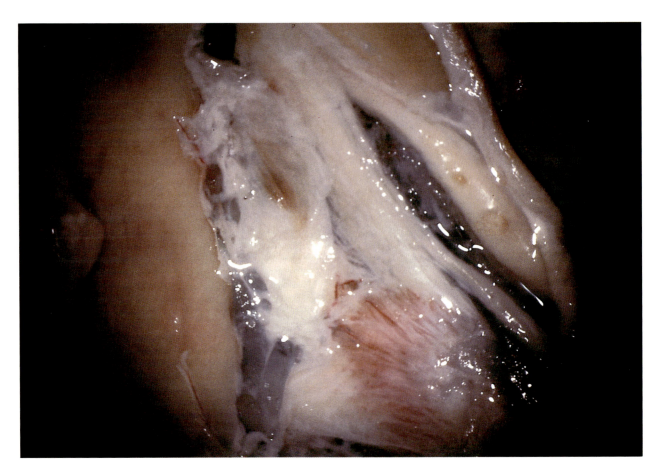

Fig. 64. Further removal of the venous jnjection from the lateral wall of the CS shows the enlarged venous bed in this area and a small entrance of the vein close to the bone at the base of the anterolateral triangle. At this point "venous blood" runs into the CS. A large amount of venous injection is seen in the paramedial triangle, in Parkinson's triangle, and over V3. The "venous blood" runs from the CS lateral and medial to the GG and the Vth nerve toward the SPS and down to the inferior petrosal sinus

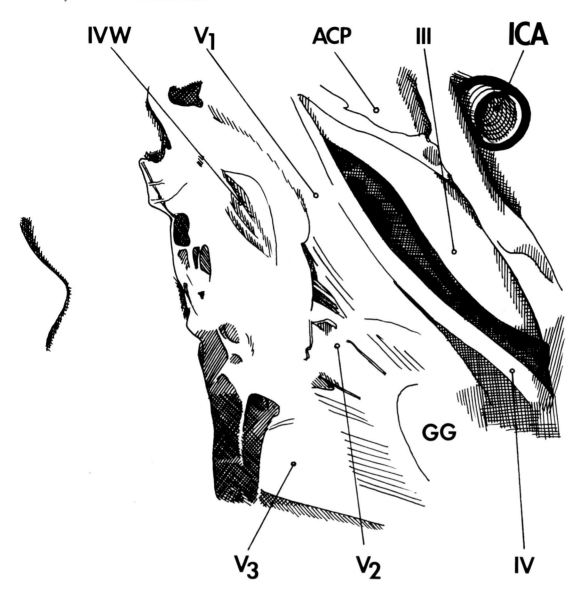

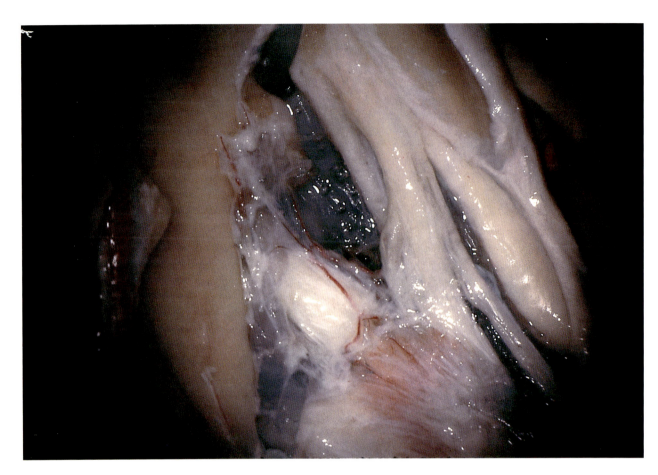

Fig. 65. Further removal of the lateral wall of the CS shows the orbital vein entering the CS through the anterolateral triangle. The anterolateral triangle is filled with the venous injection as are all the other compartments of the left CS

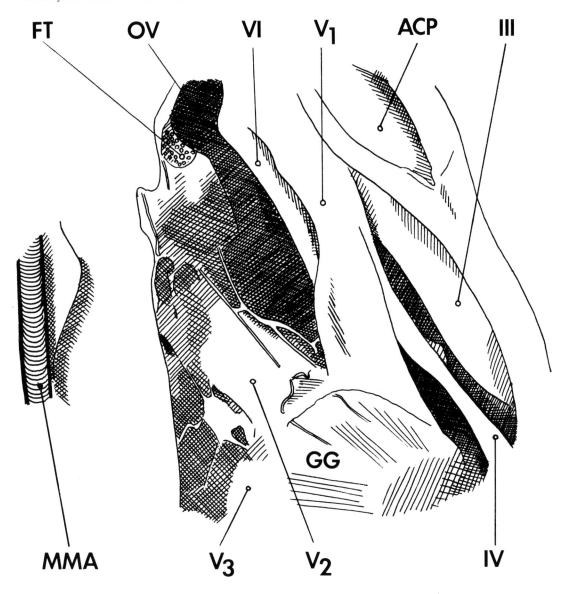

2 General approach to the cavernous sinus

The initial position of the patient is as for the pterional approach [55], the patient lying supine with head fixed in the Mayfield tripoint fixator. In order to expose the fronto-temporal region on the side of the lesion in the CS, the head is rotated by about 35 degrees in the opposite direction to the lesion (Fig. 66). The skin incision curves from the ear to the intersection of the midline with the hairline whereby the concavity of the curve faces anteriorly towards the eye (Fig. 66). The skin flap together with the subcutaneous layer is pulled down frontally over the edge of the orbit and dissected to the orbital margin (Fig. 68). The muscle flap is formed by an incision in the muscle close to its attachment to the bone, running from the junction of the zygoma and the orbital margin posteriorly to the end of the exposed muscle and along its edge caudally towards the ear (Fig. 68). The insertion of the muscle is preserved on the bone whereas the lateral part of the muscle flap is elevated and fixed with hooks laterally. Using a raspatory, periosteum is detached from the orbital margin at the corner where the zygoma and the orbital margin join (Fig. 69). Trephination is carried out in three points: at the site of the junction of the zygoma and the orbit, temporally, and fronto-temporo-parietally. The trephination hole in the front is placed so as to enable the orbit and the cranium to be opened at the same time (Fig. 70). Using an electric saw, the bone is cut between the first and the second burr hole (Fig. 70). From the first burr hole a 3 cm long cut is made lateromedially. This is done as anteriorly as possible so that the remaining orbital margin is approximately 3–4 mm wide. Following this, a semicircular cut is made from the second burr hole anteriorly, joining the previous cut (made lateromedially). The third cut is made between the third and the second burr hole. The next procedural step is to make a cut from the first burr hole downward towards the Sylvian fissure, and finally a cut is made from the third burr hole as basally as possible, temporally and postero-anteriorly. This incision ends at the very front at the sphenoid wing. The bone section is then lifted and cut away, at the sphenoid wing.

In this phase, haemostasis is performed. The most extensive bleeding usually occurs from the middle meningeal artery. Hemostasis is also effected by placing individual stay sutures between dura and bone edges. Small holes are drilled in the bone very close to the bone edge on both sides for later re-attachment of the bone flap. Matching holes are drilled at the edge of the bone flap (Fig. 71).

The opening in the orbit is enlarged and the procedure to remove the sphenoid wing is commenced (Fig. 72). The roof of the orbit is removed dorsolaterally. The sphenoid wing is removed to the lateral tip of the SOF (Fig. 73). From this point on the operation is performed under magnification. The roof of the orbit is carefully removed proceeding in the medial and lateral directions. Care must be taken so that the periosteum covering the orbital structures is not torn. Should this happen, and if fatty orbital tissue projects outward, it is cauterized and in this way retracted. Special care should be taken not to open the frontal and/or ethmoidal sinuses on the medial side whenever these are large (Fig. 73). However, if an opening should occur, care should be taken not to injure the mucous membrane. If damage to the mucosa has occurred, it is necessary to close and seal the defects in the sinus walls. Into these holes, muscle pieces are usually inserted and fixed with fibrin sealant. The sphenoid wing is resected from the SOF and from the orbital periosteum. Using a rongeur, the bone tissue is nipped away in small pieces downward toward the ACP (Fig. 74). As this process of removing the bone material approaches the peripheral end of the ON in the canal, the risk of injuring the nerve greatly increases and it is no longer possible to nip the bone tissue. Therefore at this point the bone material should be ground away. The grinding should proceed towards the centre of the ACP so that it is hollowed out (Fig. 74). Grinding is carried out also medial to the optic canal, however, with exceptional care in order not to damage the mucosa of the dorsolateral cells of the ethmoid sinus. During this grinding of the bone medial to, or lateral to the ON, and especially over it, it is of paramount importance that the drill is continuously irrigated with cold saline. In this way thermal damage to the ON will be prevented.

The process of hollowing the ACP is terminated when desired thinness of its walls is achieved; the bone is afterward broken away and removed. Such manipulation guarantees that the adjacent ON, the ICA and the structures in the SOF will not be injured. If the dorsolateral cells of the ethmoid sinus are accidentally opened and the mucous membrane damaged, the sinus must be plugged, preferably using muscle and fibrin sealant.

The ACP occasionally contains air cells from the ethmoid sinus. These air cells are usually situated under the ON, but may be above the ON. If this is so, the mucous membrane of these cells should be carefully separated from the bone and pushed back into the sinus. It is necessary to plug the opening into the sinus with muscle and fibrin sealant in order to make a watertight closure.

The ACP should never be removed by force and without hollowing it out initially. If attempts are made to remove it in one piece, the nerves in the SOF or the ICA or the ON will almost certainly be injured. It follows that the only correct procedure is to remove the ACP and the structures surrounding the ON gradually and meticulously (Fig. 75). When complete removal of the ACP is accomplished and the optic canal opened on its lateral, proximal and medial sides, complete hemostasis is performed. At this stage it must be verified that the sinuses have not been opened and that it will be possible to displace the ON in a transverse direction (Fig. 76). Usually no bleeding occurs in the bed of the previously removed ACP; however, there may sometimes be some bleeding at the very tip where it projects into the CS. When such bleeding occurs, it is stopped with a small piece of Surgicel packed into this opening. Excessive coagulation should be avoided particularly on the surface of the intracavernous ICA and, even more importantly, where the IIIrd nerve runs under the membrane and also in the immediate vicinity of the IVth and V1 nerves. Coagulation should be reduced to the minimum on the dura above the ON as well (Fig. 76).

The orbital wall is also removed posterolateral to the SOF down to the foramen rotundum. The bone peripheral to the foramen rotundum is ground away to give adequate exposure of V2 in the canal. In this way an important landmark is made which can be used later, if necessary, when the dura is opened, for following V2 from the periphery centrally toward the GG.

When the orbit has been exposed in its entirety – the orbital wall removed from the dorsal and lateral sides – and when the ON and V2 in the canal have been exposed, the operating table is rotated in the opposite direction to the pathology until the position 1+ is reached (Fig. 67). The dura is now peeled away from the bone using a subtemporal approach. The middle meningeal artery and the foramen spinosum are visualized. The dura is removed also from the petrous bone, special care being taken of the greater petrosal nerve which must be divided to prevent injury to the VIIth cranial nerve. This process of peeling the dura from the bone proceeds all the way to the Vth cranial nerve. The middle meningeal artery is coagulated and divided just in front of the foramen spinosum which is then packed with a piece of Surgicel and sealed with bone wax. Following this, the drilling of the bone begins approximately 5–6 mm medially from the foramen spinosum and just behind the dorsal aspect of the GG and V3. At this point, the tensor tympani is encountered which is a landmark for the Eustachian tube. Once the position of the tensor tympani is established, the drilling is continued somewhat more medially, away from this muscle and from the Eustachian tube. The drilling process is carried out very carefully, with the drill bit constantly irrigated with saline solution. After a few revolutions of the drill, the ICA in the petrous bone can be visualized. This portion of the ICA frequently lies uncovered by bone. In such cases, the whole procedure is much easier to perform. Whether or not this is so, however, the edges of the bone are still ground away in order to improve the operative exposure of the ICA. Using a dissector, the ICA should be dissected from the inside surface of the canal so that it is possible to place two temporary clips on it. All this preparation is imperative before opening the dura. The exposure of the ICA in the canal is required for other reasons in addition to placement of temporary clips; potential grafting of the ICA from the segment in the petrous bone to the segment of its anterior loop or intradurally may be necessary, or, a definitive occlusion of the artery may be necessary if the ICA can be neither preserved nor grafted at this site.

After the ON in the canal, the anterior loop of the ICA in the anteromedial triangle, V2 in the canal peripheral to the foramen rotundum, and the ICA in the petrous bone have been exposed, an incision in the dura is made (Fig. 82). The incision begins approximately 2 cm from the lateral tip of the SOF and proceeds toward this tip. Before the lateral tip of the SOF is reached, one arm of the incision is made on the medial side and the other on the lateral side of the SOF itself. The incision medial to the SOF is directed downward, to the base of the previously removed ACP, then it turns medially for 90 degrees and the dura is incised across the ON. A band of dura approximately 2–3 mm wide remains to allow for watertight reconstruction of the dura at the end of the operation. The lateral incision encircles the CS so that about 2–3 mm of the dura is left in a semicircle from the SOF and across V2 in front of the foramen rotundum. The incision afterwards runs laterodorsally across V3 where again a 2–3 mm band of dura remains at the edge of the CS. The dura is also incised strictly dorsally, parallel to V3 on the dorsal side of the GG. The dural flap covering the temporal and frontal lobes is left to protect the brain tissue when it is retracted by a spatula. It has been found that such protection of brain tissue has advantages over any other material placed directly on the cortex.

Only when the dura has been opened, can the first CSF be aspirated. In the procedures in the CS, lumbar drainage should never be used. It is believed that maintenance of CSF volume and dural integrity during the removal and drilling of the bone epidurally constitute the best shield against possible trauma. For this reason also, the patients are never dehydrated intraoperatively. Hypotension, hypothermy, and extracorporeal circulation also should not be used.

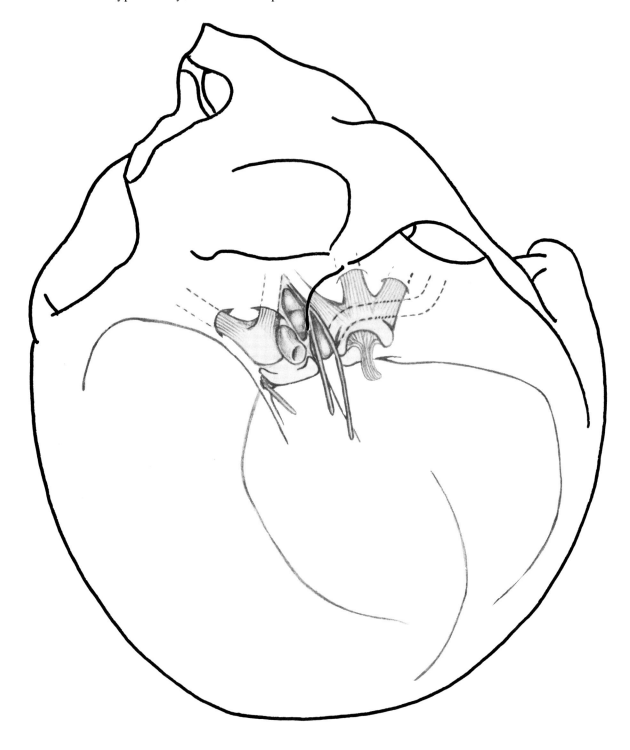

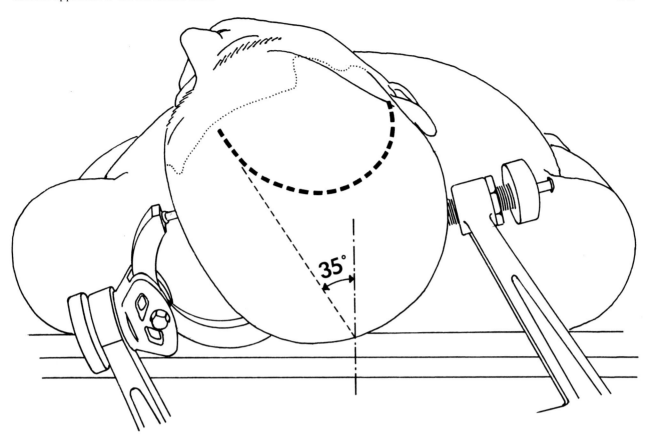

Fig. 66. The initial position of the patient's head is shown. The head is fixed in the Mayfield tripoint fixator. The ideal rotation of the head in the opposite direction to the lesion in the CS is about 35°. While the body of the patient is in the supine position, further rotation in the same direction would cause twisting of the neck and hence possible impairment of venous drainage from the head. For that reason, it is of paramount importance to ensure that the veins in the neck are not stretched or twisted, and that the position of the head in relation to the position of the body is not changed throughout the operation. The same also applies to deflexion of the head. Initially, the head is positioned so that the junction point of the zygomatic arch and the orbital rim is the highest point. In this way, both the rotation and tilting of the head are determined. When any other positioning of the head is required during surgery, it can be easily and safely achieved by rotation of the table to the left or to the right, with or without tilting of the table. In this way the initial position of the head in relation to the initial position of the body will remain unchanged. This will ensure normal venous drainage from the brain during surgery, which will result in a slack brain providing proper neuroanaesthesia and surgical handling of the brain tissue

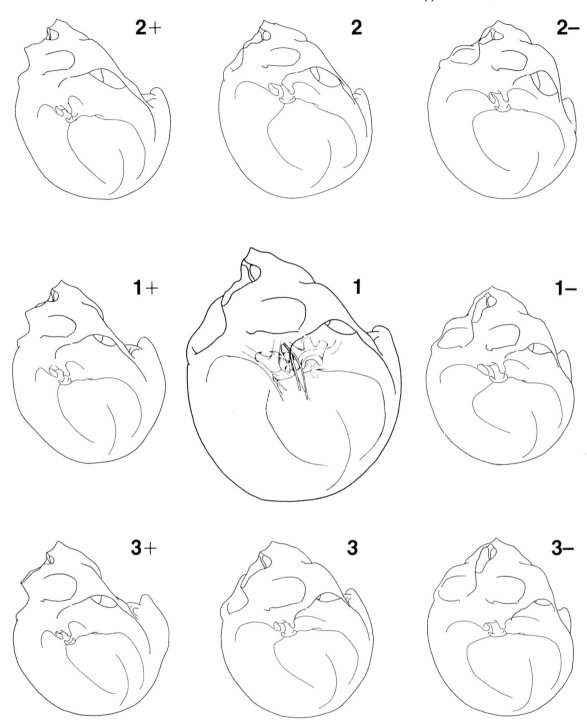

Fig. 67. Nine principal positions of the head are shown. Rotating the table from the initial position 1, but without tilting, lateral position 1+ and anteroposterior position 1– can be reached. With tilting of the table in the direction "head up", positions 2, 2+, and 2– can be reached. With tilting of the table in the direction "head down", positions 3, 3+ and 3– can be reached. It goes without saying that with appropriate positioning of the head, the individual structures in and around the CS can be reached with minimal retraction of the brain. Proper positioning of the head throughout the operation requires the ability to continuously change the position and contributes greatly to the success of the operation

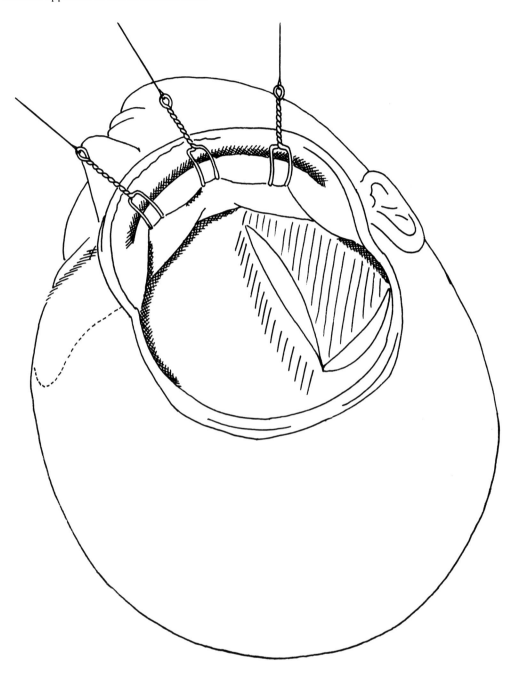

Fig. 68. The skin flap together with the subcutaneous tissue has been retracted and positioned frontotemporally over the eye. The skin flap is fixed with fish hooks so that the junction point of the zygomatic arch and the orbital arch is exposed. The temporal muscle is incised from the junction point of the zygomatic arch and orbital arch in a posterior direction so that the insertion of the temporal muscle is left in place thus enabling the surgeon to perform appropriate fixation of the temporal muscle to the bone at the end of the operation. Posteriorly, the temporal muscle is incised along the direction of muscle fibers towards the ear

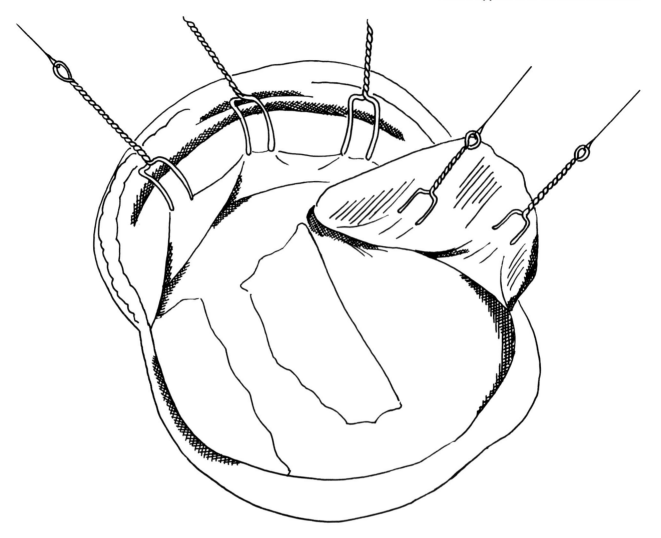

Fig. 69. The muscle flap has been separated from the temporal bone, lifted and fixed with a pair of fish hooks in a lateral direction. Such a positioning of the muscle flap allows good access to the point of junction of the zygomatic arch with the orbital arch. Insertion of the temporal muscle is left in place. The periosteum of the frontal bone is cut and separated

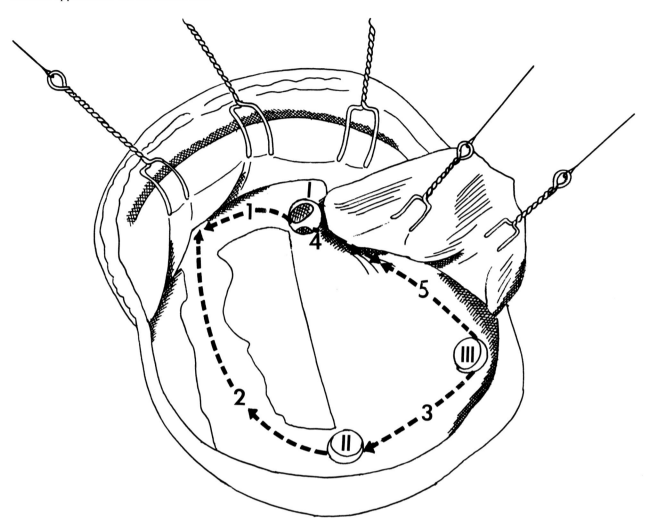

Fig. 70. The position of the head is unchanged. With the craniotome 3 burr holes (*I–III*) have been performed. The broken line with the arrows indicates the positioning of the bone cut. *1–5* Indicate the sequence of the bone cuts. Note: The burr hole I has been placed posterior to the junction point of the zygomatic and orbital arches for cosmetic reasons and performed in such a direction that the orbit and the endocranium have been opened simultaneously

OR   ORBIT   SW   TM

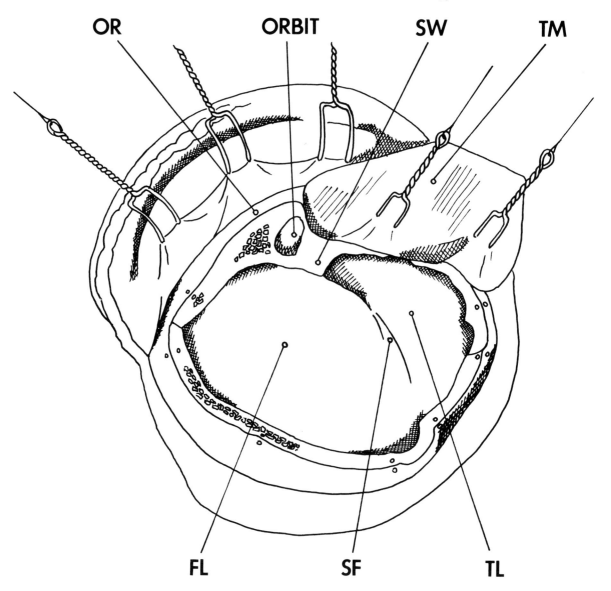

FL   SF   TL

Fig. 71. The frontotemporal bone flap has been lifted and the dura over the frontal and temporal lobes exposed. The lateral part of the sphenoid wing and the orbital rim have been exposed and the orbit opened. Holes into the bone on the corresponding opposite points along the bone cut have been made enabling proper fixation of the bone flap at the end of the operation

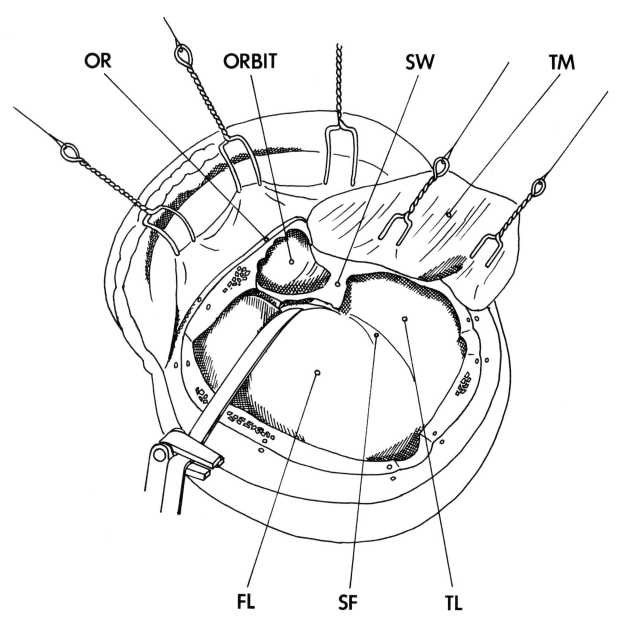

Fig. 72. The head is still in the initial position. The orbit has been further unroofed. From the intracranial side the dura is gently removed from the roof of the orbit. From the intraorbital side, the periosteum is also gently removed from the roof of the orbit. Only when the roof of the orbit is free of tissue from the intraorbital and intracranial sides can the bone be removed. For this reason, unroofing of the orbit must be performed under magnification. The dura should be preserved intact so that retraction of the dura does not damage the brain

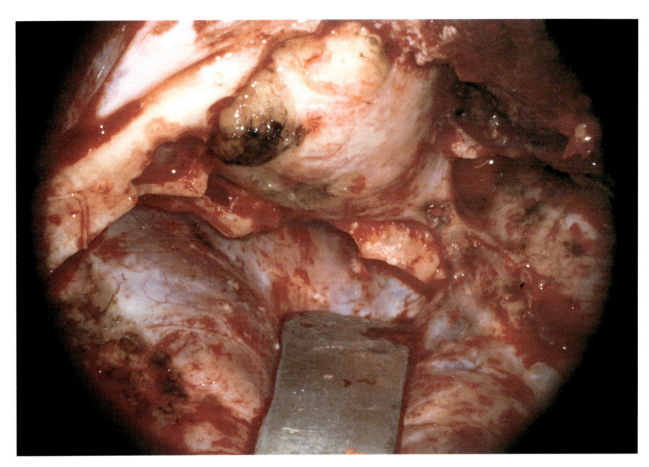

Fig. 73. The head is in the position 2 – (Fig. 67). Further removal of the roof of the orbit on the anterior and posterior sides of the SOF has been performed. The dura running from the temporal lobe through the SOF into the orbit has been exposed. On the medial side the frontal sinus has been accidentally opened during removal of the roof of the orbit. Regardless of the integrity of the mucous membrane the frontal sinus should be properly closed with pieces of muscle and fibrin glue at the end of the operation to prevent CSF leakage

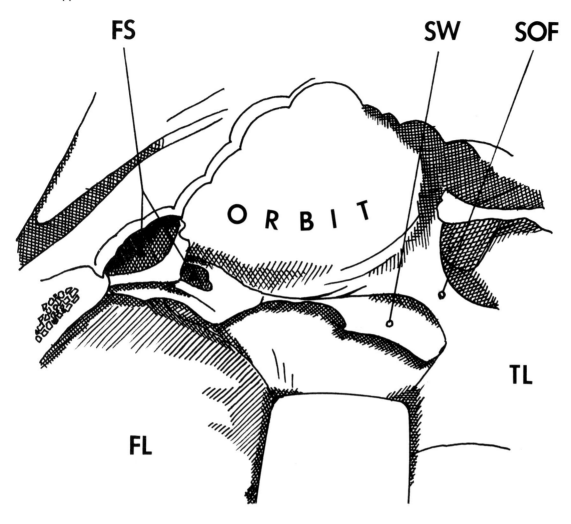

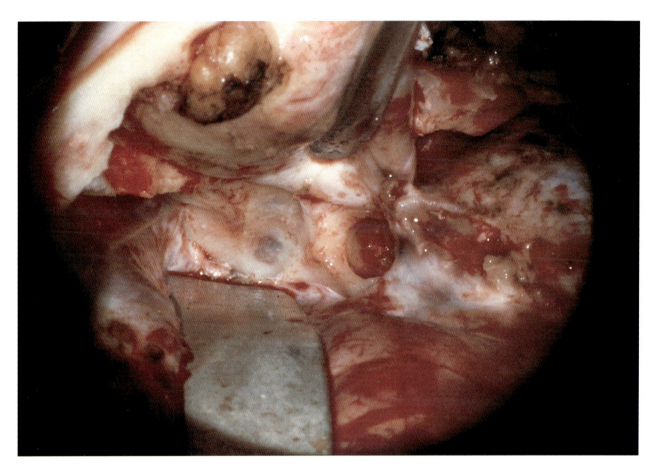

Fig. 74. The sphenoid wing has been removed further toward the ACP. The ACP itself has been hollowed out already. The roof of the orbit has been removed completely down to the optic canal. The dorsal wall of the optic canal has been partially removed and the dura propria visualized. On the medial aspect of the ON, the bone has been drilled off and the mucous membrane of the ethmoid sinus can be traced through the thin bony layer overlying it. Slight retraction of the orbital compartments in an anterolateral direction is necessary to visualize the peripheral end of the optic canal. Attention should be paid to the periosteum covering the orbital tissue so that it is preserved intact

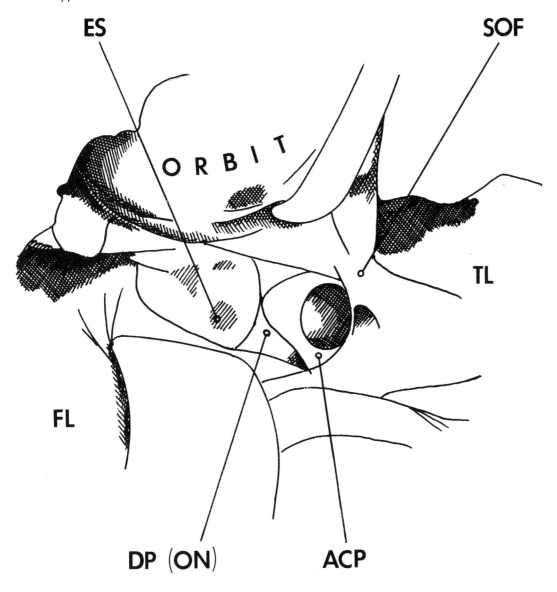

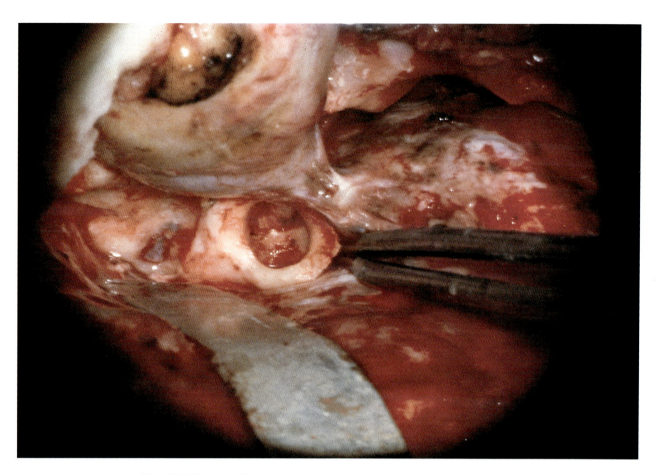

Fig. 75. The head is placed in the position 2– (Fig. 67), which gives an appropriate view toward the ACP. The ACP has been drilled out from inside and then dissected and mobilized from the medial side of the dura covering the neural structures running from the CS through the SOF to the orbit. The ACP is usually firmly attached to the surrounding dura, and should never be forcibly pulled out. It is much safer to drill the bulk of the bone from inside toward the periphery unless the walls of the ACP are thin, in which case they can easily be separated from the dura and gently removed with pituitary forceps. Continuous irrigation is mandatory while drilling the ACP and the walls of the optic canal. Heat injury to the ON and to the IIIrd, IVth, and V1 nerves is very likely if cooling of the drill bit by continuous irrigation is not carried out. On the medial side of the optic canal, the ethmoid sinus has been opened. It goes without saying that irrespective of the integrity of the mucous membrane of the bony sinus, at the end of the operation it must be closed watertightly with pieces of muscle and fibrin glue to prevent CSF leakage

ES

SOF

O R B I T

TL

FL

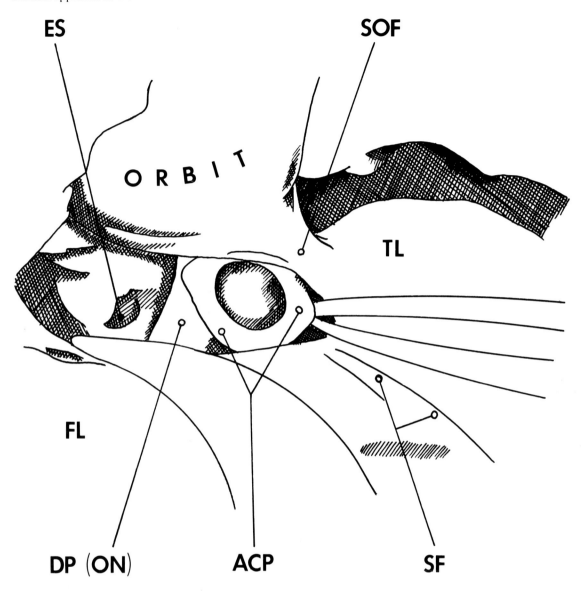

DP (ON)   **ACP**   **SF**

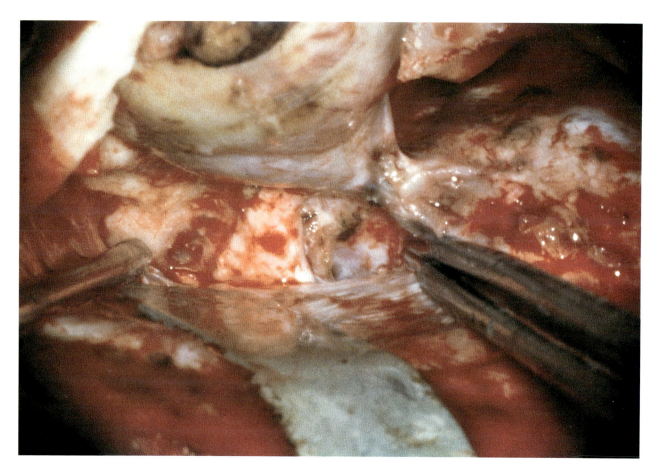

Fig. 76. The orbit has been unroofed to a sufficient extent in the anterolateral region, medial and lateral to the SOF. The optic canal has been opened from its medial, dorsal and lateral sides. The dura propria covering the ON is shown from the dura to the orbital tissue. The ACP has been completely removed. The anterior loop of the ICA can be traced through the thin membrane covering the anterior loop of the ICA from the distal dural ring to the proximal ring. The mucous membrane of the ethmoid sinus medial to the optic canal has been exposed. The dura covering the frontal and temporal lobes is still intact. The bone on the dorsal aspect of the SOF toward the foramen rotundum has been removed

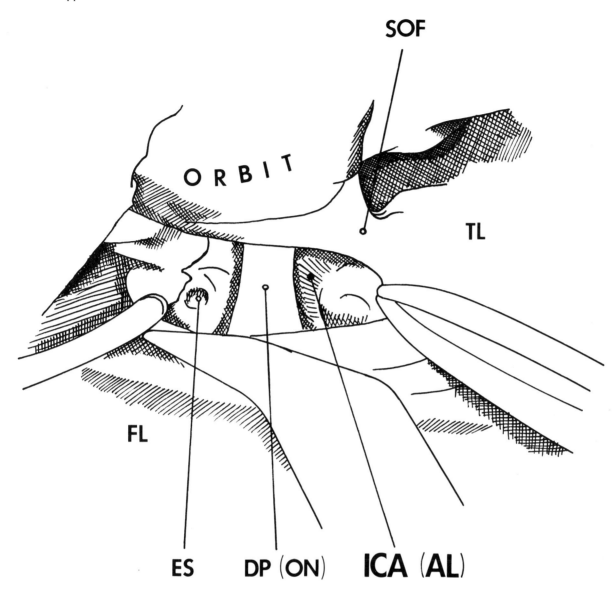

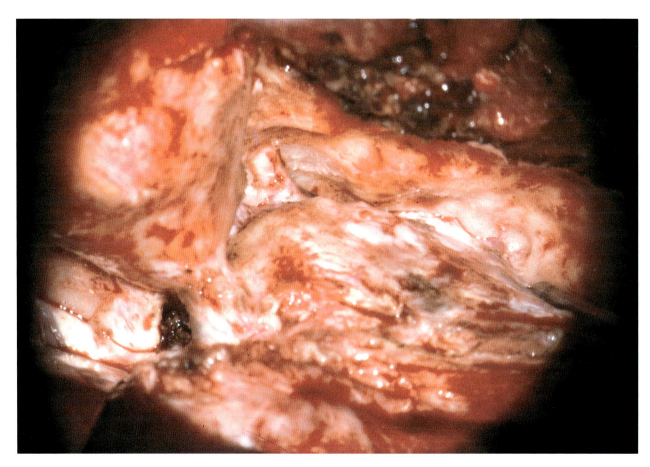

Fig. 77. The position of the head is the initial position according to the rotation but with the "head up" tilting of the table which offers much better visualization toward the foramen rotundum. The bone around V2 peripheral to the foramen rotundum has been removed and approximately 1 cm of V2 in the canal has been dissected. The unroofing of V2 in the canal peripheral to the foramen rotundum is necessary for dissection of V2 in a retrograde direction, i. e. from the periphery toward the GG. From V1 the unroofed orbital tissue covered by periosteum, the dura running between the temporal lobe and the orbit, and the dura propria covering the ON in the whole length of its course through the optic canal, are shown. The anteromedial triangle is packed with Surgicel. On the lateral side of V2 the foramen ovale and middle meningeal artery can be seen

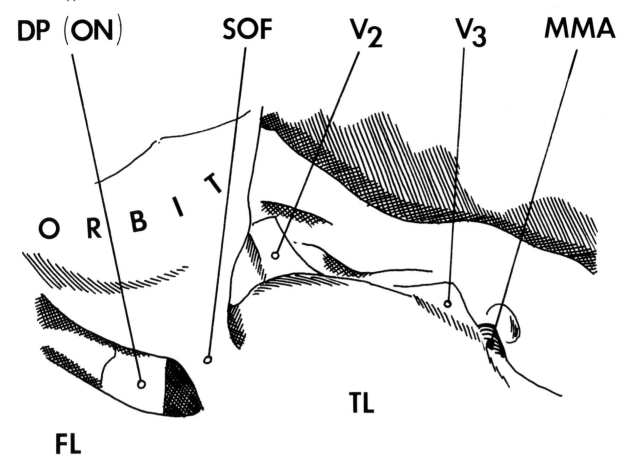

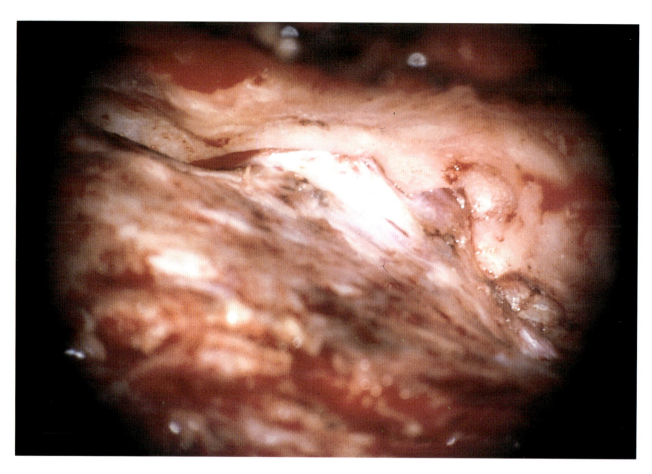

Fig. 78. The head is in the position 2+ (Fig. 67). This position offers a lateral subtemporal approach toward the foramen rotundum and foramen spinosum. The middle meningeal artery has been dissected and shown at the exit point from the foramen spinosum. The foramen ovale with V3 covered by the dura is shown

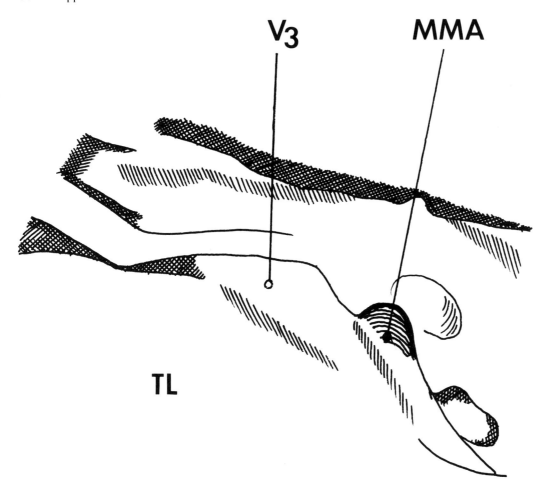

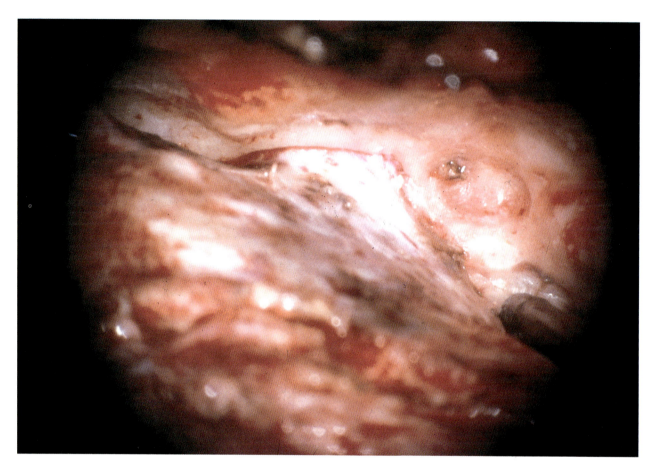

Fig. 79. The middle meningeal artery has been dissected and cut close to the foramen spinosum. The proximal stump of the middle meningeal artery has been coagulated and pushed into the foramen spinosum. The bone posterior to the foramen spinosum has been drilled off. V3 covered with dura is seen at the entry point into the foramen ovale. The head is in the position 2+ (Fig. 67) which allows for a subtemporal lateral approach

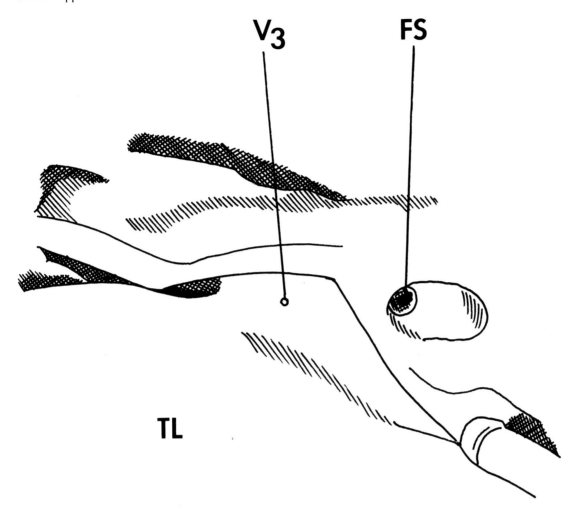

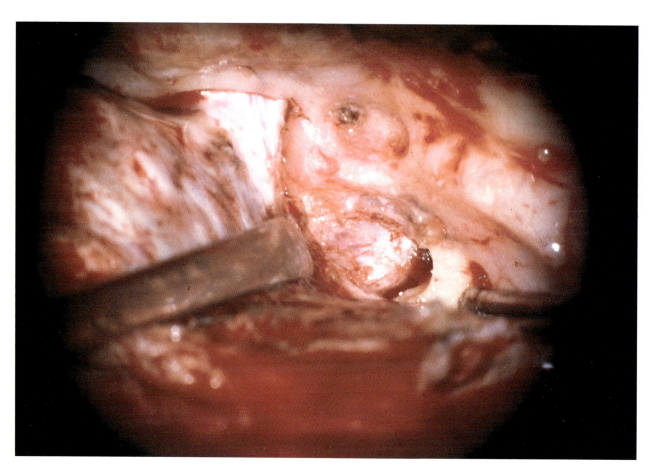

Fig. 80. The head is in the position 2+ (Fig. 67). The middle meningeal artery has been dissected, cut and coagulated. The bone over the ICA in the posterolateral triangle has been drilled off and the artery can be seen at its posterior loop. The greater petrosal nerve has been cut. The tensor tympani muscle has been exposed lateral to the ICA. V3 covered with dura is retracted anteriorly

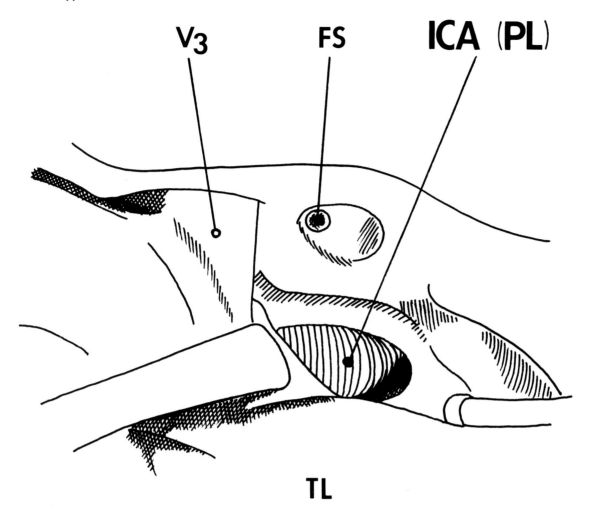

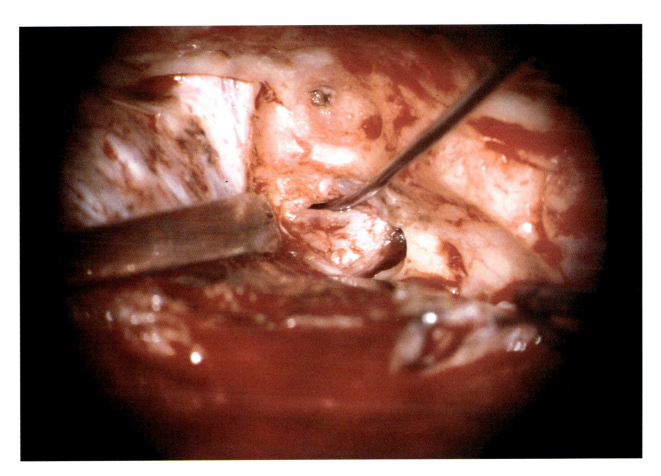

Fig. 81. The head is in the position 2+ (Fig. 67). Further dissection of the posterior loop of the ICA in the petrous bone has been performed and the artery dissected from the bony walls of the canal in its whole circumference. Only when the ICA has been dissected from the bone can a temporary clip be properly placed on it. Whereas, if the artery has not been completely dissected from the bone, a temporary clip will not occlude the artery completely . On the other hand, it is necessary to dissect at least a length of 2 cm of the ICA in order to provide a good proximal stump for reconstruction of the ICA when necessary. Further retraction of V3 over the dura in an anterior direction enables further dissection of the ICA in the canal toward the foramen lacerum. V3 covered with dura cannot be damaged while being retracted if the dura is intact

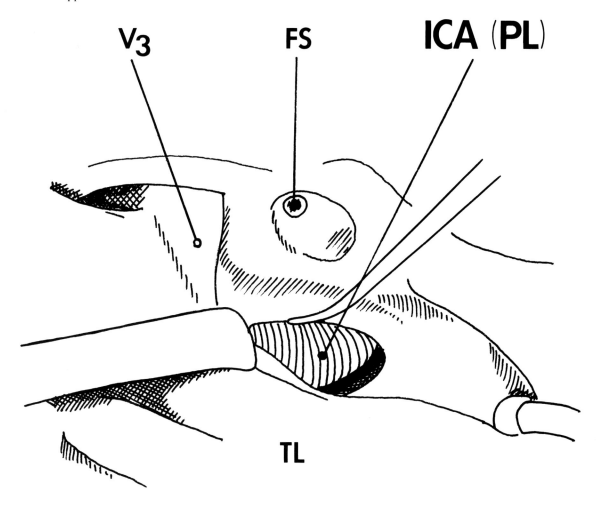

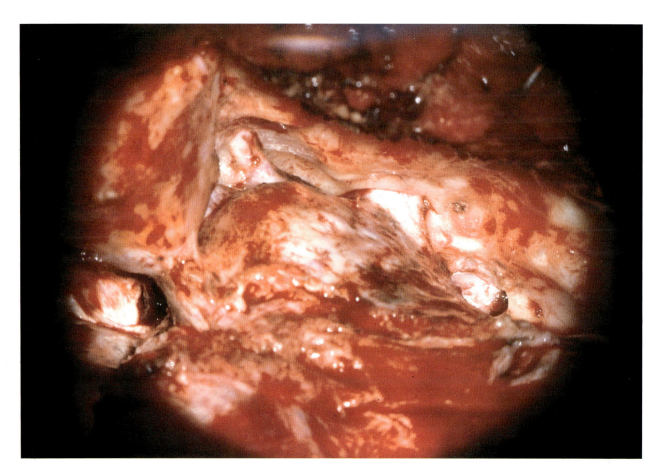

Fig. 82. The head is in the position 2 (Fig. 67). The epidural stage of the operation for all intracavernous pathology has now been completed. The dura has not been damaged and the CSF has not been removed neither on purpose nor accidentally. The ON covered with dura propria, anteromedial triangle, dura running from the temporal lobe to the orbit, V1 in the canal peripheral to the foramen rotundum, V3 entering the foramen ovale, foramen spinosum with the proximal stump of the middle meningeal artery and the ICA in the canal of the petrous bone, as well as the dura over the temporal lobe and the periosteum covering the orbital structures, are sufficiently exposed. Only after such a complete epidural exposure of the structures can the dura be incised. The incision of the dura runs along the Sylvian fissure toward the lateral tip of the SOF, extending toward the anteromedial triangle. When it reaches the base of the triangle it turns medially over the ICA and over the ON. The other arm of the Y-shaped incision runs lateral to the SOF and curves around the CS lateral to V1, V2, V3 and over the ICA where it ends. Such a dural incision enables watertight closure of the dura at the end of the operation. At the same time the dural flaps are used instead of cotton pads to protect the surface of the brain while retracting it with spatulas

ON   **SOF**   **V₂**   **V₃**   **FS**   **ICA (PL)**

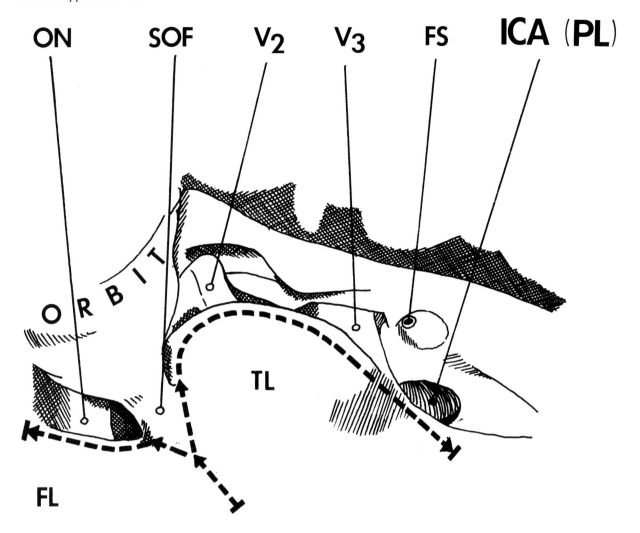

ORBIT

TL

FL

3.1 Combined epi- and subdural approach to carotid ophthalmic aneurysms

Surgery of carotid ophthalmic aneurysms, which was until recently a very demanding procedure, has become much safer and easier to perform by employing the combined epi- and subdural approach [8]. In this procedure a standard pterional craniotomy [55, 56] is used, following this is removal of the orbital roof together with the sphenoid wing and the ACP. Then the proximal, medial, and lateral part of the wall of the optic canal are removed to give the operative exposure of the ON from the dura to the entry point into the intraorbital tissue, in its entire segment in the optic canal. The orbital roof is removed on the anterior side of the SOF, as well as on its dorsal side. For this type of aneurysm it is enough if the anterior loop of the ICA in the anteromedial triangle is exposed. Therefore, it is not necessary to explore the ICA in the carotid canal in the petrous bone through the posterolateral triangle. The dissection of the ICA in the anteromedial triangle is essential and must be completed before the dissection of the aneurysm itself is commenced. With this type of aneurysm it is important that the dura is not damaged while operating epidurally and removing the bone. In addition, this is imperative when dealing with large or giant carotid ophthalmic aneurysms which are not thrombosed. Equally important is that the intradural pressure is not lowered by lumbar drainage which is contraindicated in this type of surgery. Maintaining the normal cerebrospinal fluid quantity and pressure by preserving the intact dura is the best protection of the underlying aneurysm, the brain, and the neural structures from mechanical injury during the drilling of the ACP. Care must be taken because the ACP is tightly attached to the dura.

It cannot be emphasized enough that it is of utmost importance that the drill is constantly irrigated during the drilling of the bone around the ON. The ON is quite well protected from mechanical drilling damage by its dural sheath. Care is required, however, during the operation to avoid accidental injury to the ON. More importantly, it must be realized that the ON can be damaged by the heat generated during the drilling of the bone. Therefore, the drill tip must be constantly bathed with saline solution.

As opposed to long periods of drilling, very short drilling periods are used each time followed by an examination of the thickness of the underlying layer of the bone. These short periods of drilling should consist of only a few revolutions of the drill bit. This same cautious procedure must be performed when drilling the bone on the medial aspect of the optic canal where the drill can easily slip into the lateral dorsal cells of the ethmoid sinus with resultant damage to the mucous membrane.

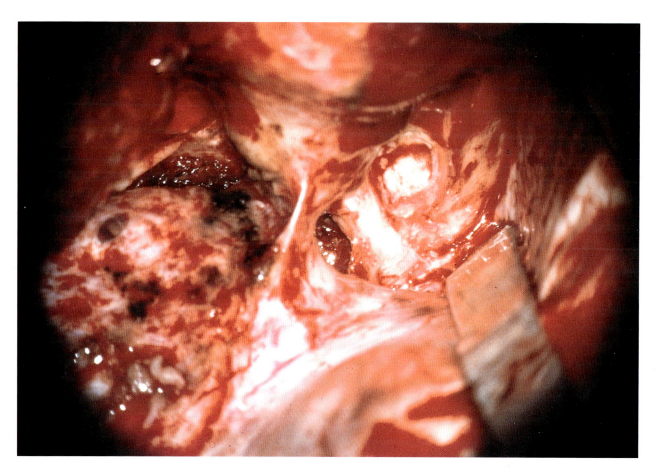

Fig. 83. The completed first phase of the combined epi- and subdural approach to the carotid ophthalmic aneurysm is presented. The unroofed orbit, the SOF, the dura covering the temporal and frontal lobe, and the ON covered by dura propria are shown. Between the ON and the SOF, the ICA can be seen running in a semicircular path. It can be noticed that the artery is still covered by a fibrous membrane. The ACP is completely removed. In addition, it can be seen that the thin bone wall between the ICA and the ON has been removed. On the medial side of the ON, the exposed mucous membrane of the dorsal lateral cells of the ethmoid sinus can be seen. The mucous membrane is preserved intact

While drilling the lateral wall of the optic canal, care should be taken not to damage the wall of either the sphenoid sinus or the ICA.

Intraoperative views from the opening of the dura to clipping of a **left** sided large carotid ophthalmic aneurysm are shown in Figs. 83–90.

SOF

ES

ORBIT

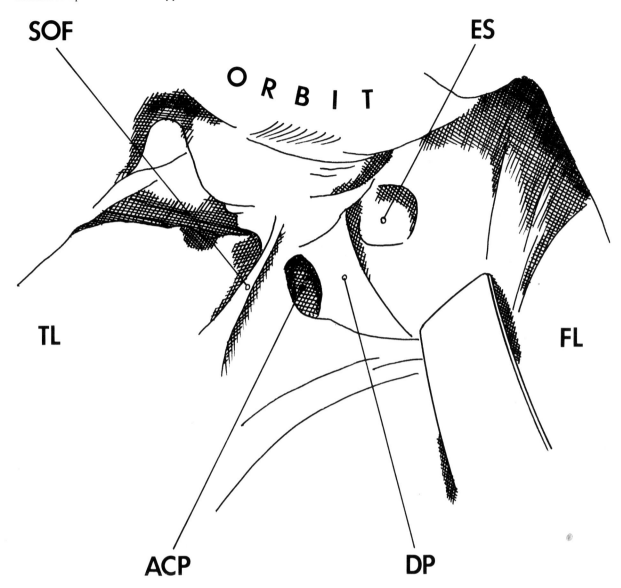

TL

FL

ACP

DP

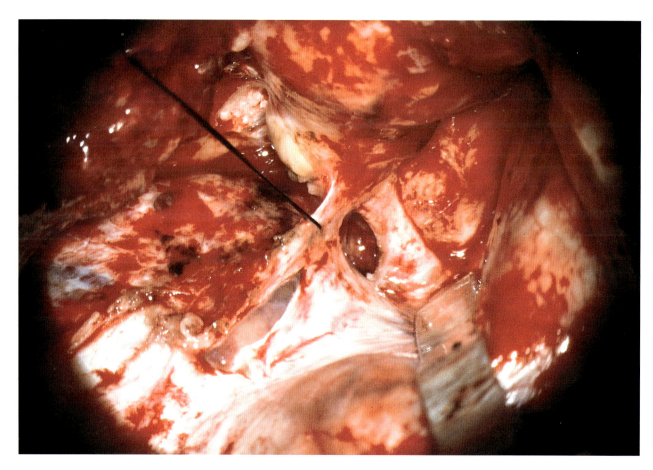

Fig. 84. Following complete removal of the whole sphenoid wing together with the ACP
and complete exposure of the ON in its entire length in the optic canal, the second step of
the operation is started. First, the lateral tip of the SOF is fixed with a stay suture. The
incision into the dura is made along the Sylvian fissure, 2 cm from the lateral tip of the SOF

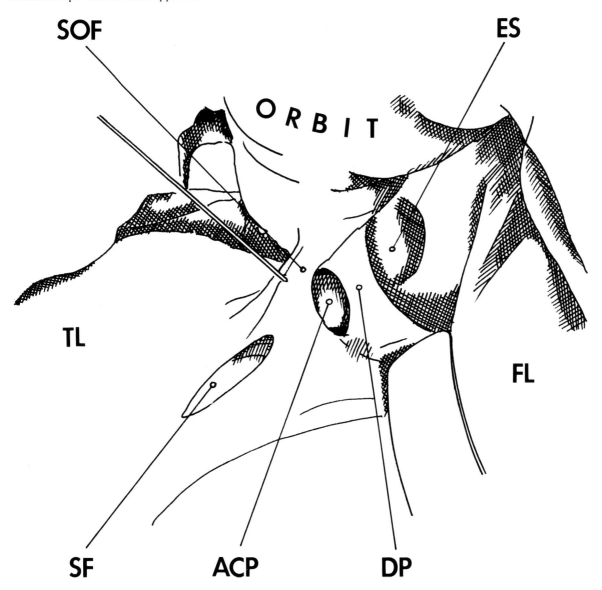

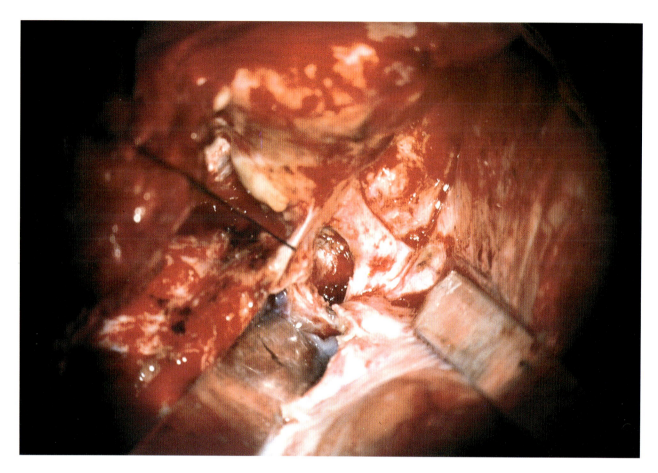

Fig. 85. The incision of the dura is made from the lateral tip of the SOF toward the ON, medial to the SOF to the original position of the ACP and to the base of the anteromedial triangle. The incision is made medially enough in order to preserve an adequate width of the dura along the SOF which facilitates watertight closure of the dura at the end of the operation. When the incision of the dura intersects a line connecting the entry points of the ON and the IIIrd nerve into the optic canal and into the lateral wall of the CS respectively, it turns in a medial direction

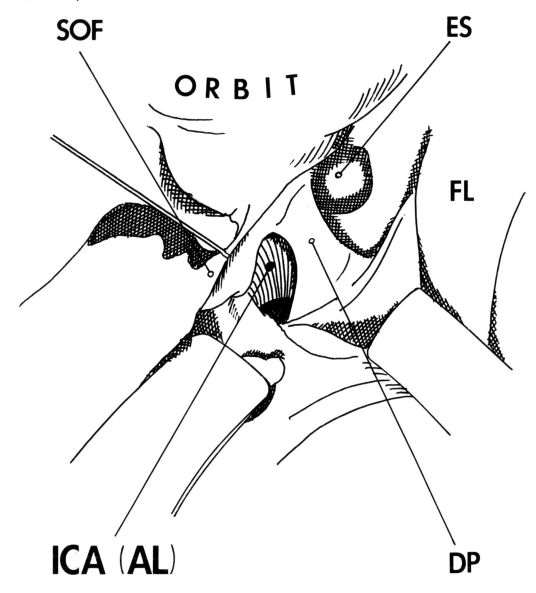

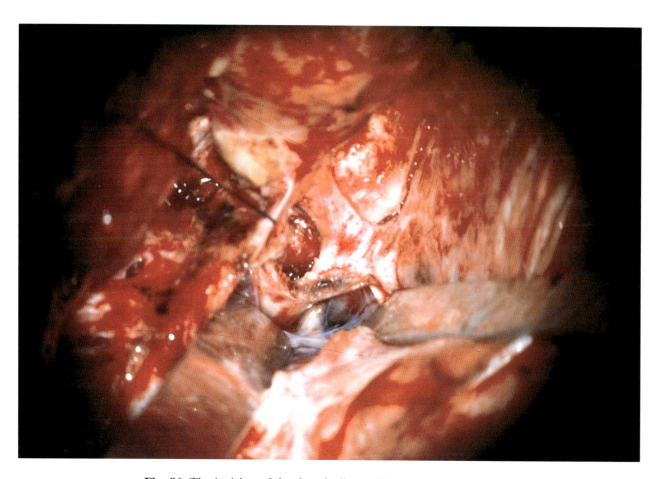

Fig. 86. The incision of the dura is directed downward and medially over the ICA toward the ON. Approximately 2–3 mm of the dural ring around the ICA is left in place. The dura is continued to be cut more medially over the ON somewhat dorsal to the entry point of the ON into the dural sleeve of the dura propria which guides the ON from the intracranial to the intraorbital end. Then the incision of the dura in a transverse direction is made in such a way that a few millimeters of the dura are preserved on the base over the ON. This strip of the dura will later facilitate watertight closure. The incision of the dura from the lateral aspect across the ICA and over displaced and usually deformed ON must be carefully made in order that, first, the ICA is not damaged and, secondly, that the aneurysm and the ON are also not injured. Note the anterior loop of the ICA in the anteromedial triangle, the ICA intradurally, the aneurysm under the ON, and the lateral edge of the ON which is markedly proximally displaced and stretched over the aneurysm

ICA (AL)   DP (ON)   ES

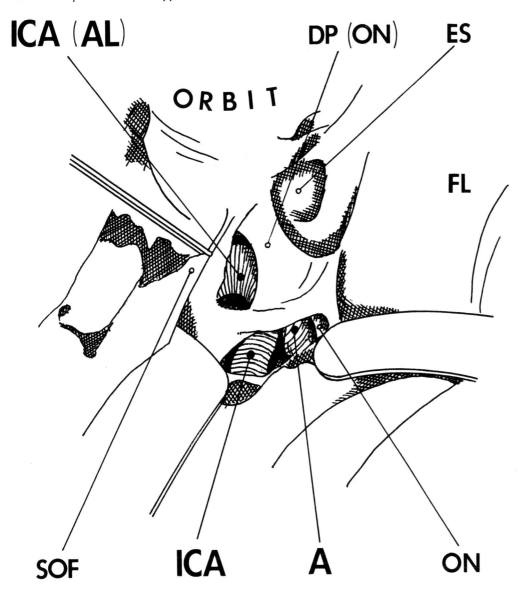

ORBIT   FL

SOF   ICA   A   ON

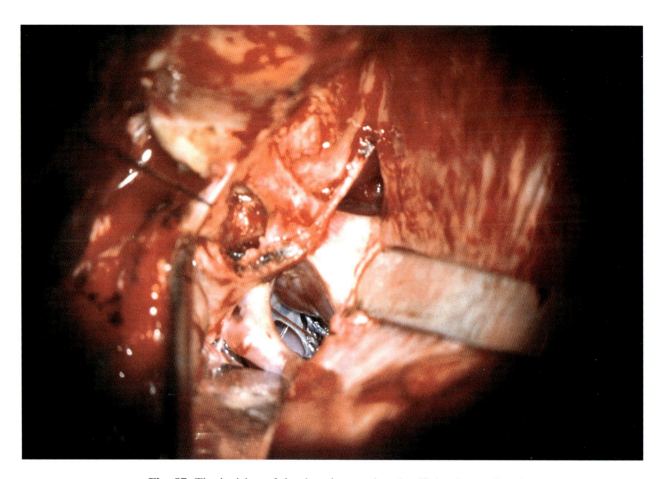

Fig. 87. The incision of the dura is completed sufficiently to allow for combined epi- and subdural approach to the carotid ophthalmic artery aneurysm. At this point the ICA and the ACoA intradurally are exposed. Transversely across the longitudinal axis of the ICA and across the ON a narrow band of the dura is left in place. The ON is seen both intradurally and extradurally (where it is covered with dura propria). The intradural portion of the ON is compressed from below and stretched over the large aneurysm. The dural flap which was made with the cut described in Figs. 84–87 serves as protection for the brain. The dura which is to be lifted, is placed over the brain so that it is not necessary to use cotton or any other material over the brain cortex. It is believed that this method provides the most natural protection against mechanical injury to the brain. The frontal lobe is carefully retracted across the dura, thus exposing the ICA from the aneurysm to the bifurcation into the ACA and MCA. In the same way, the markedly changed ON is exposed to the point of its transition to the optic tract laterally, and to the optic chiasm medially. Under the ON, the aneurysm is visualized on both the lateral and medial sides of the left ON

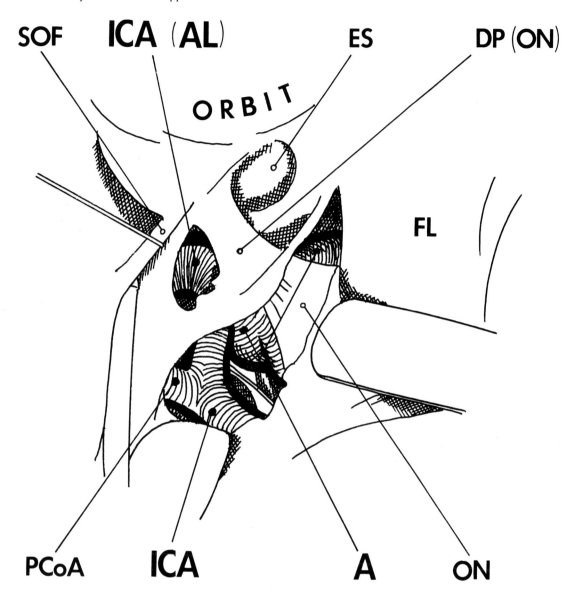

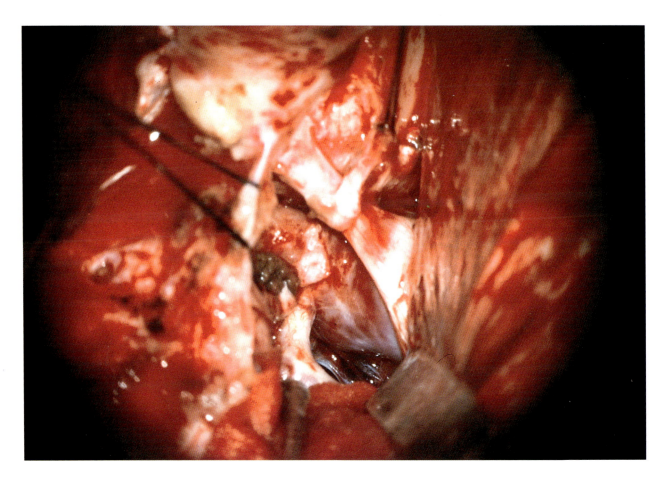

Fig. 88. Only when the ICA is exposed in the anteromedial triangle proximal to the ophthalmic artery and intrathecally distal to the aneurysm sufficiently for temporary clipping, can dissection of the neck of the aneurysm be started. First, the dural ring around the ICA is cut and fixed medially over the ON. The dural ring is also cut in a lateral direction toward the IIIrd nerve and the PCP. When the exposure of the neck of the aneurysm and its relationship to the ophthalmic artery is hampered by partial opening of the dural ring around the ICA, the opening should be continued circumferentially around the ICA so that the latter can be completely mobilized. The ICA is followed in the proximal direction and is dissected from the wall of the bone anteriorly and medially. Posteriorly and laterally in the concavity of the anterior loop of the ICA, the membrane which covers the ICA is cut and Surgicel is placed around the artery on both sides. In this way, a segment of the ICA is mobilized proximally from the dural ring in the anteromedial triangle and this allows not only placement of a temporary clip proximal to the ophthalmic artery and aneurysm, but also displacement of the ICA to a greater extent from the medial to the lateral direction. At the same time, the mobilization of the ICA proximal to the ophthalmic artery allows an approach with the clip from the proximal direction and medial to the ophthalmic artery to the neck of the aneurysm when necessary. In most cases, the clip can be placed over the neck of the aneurysm from the peripheral intrathecal side toward the inferomedial aspect of the ICA extradurally in the anteromedial triangle hence the dural ring around the ICA obstructs no longer the proper placement of the blades of the clip. If a clip cannot be placed from either direction on the neck of the aneurysm, temporary clips are placed proximal and distal to the aneurysm, the aneurysm is resected,

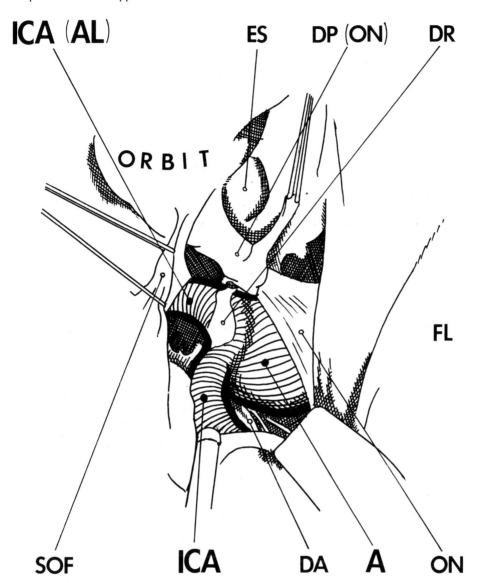

and the wall of the ICA reconstructed by interrupted sutures. Such reconstruction of the ICA wall is only possible when sufficient rotation of the ICA around the longitudinal axis is provided

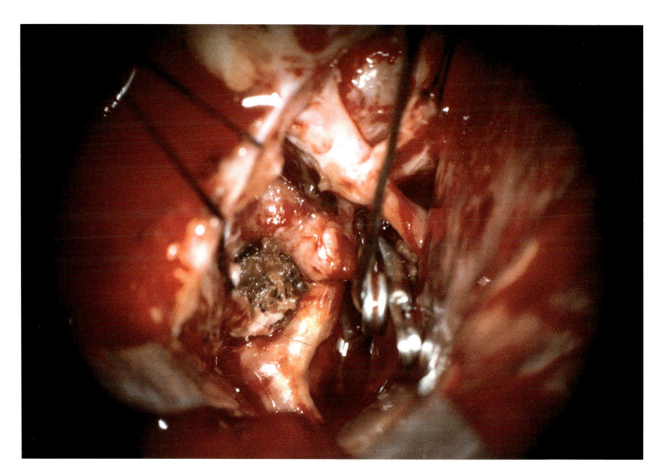

Fig. 89. Two clips are seen on the neck of the aneurysm. The aneurysm is slack as the blood has been aspirated from the sac. The ON is no longer compressed from the inferior aspect. The ophthalmic artery is shown and is fully preserved. The ICA distal to the aneurysm is kinked, however, because of revision of the position of the clips, which are held medially from the ICA with the dissector. The blades of the clips are placed across the whole width of the neck of the aneurysm so that the ophthalmic artery is free and patent as well as the ICA

SOF   ICA (AL)   DP (ON)   ES   OA

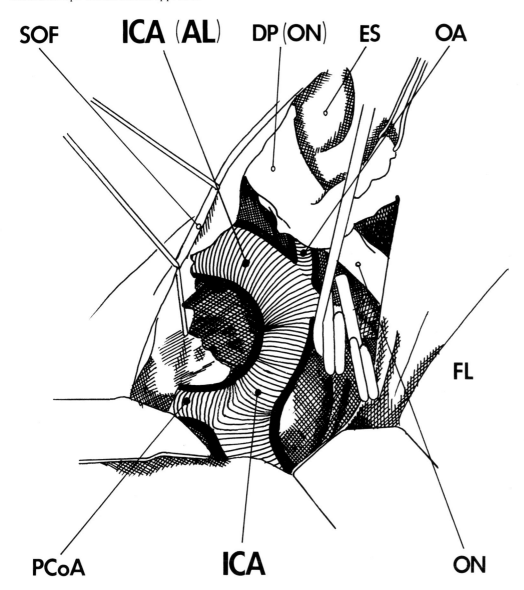

PCoA   ICA   ON

FL

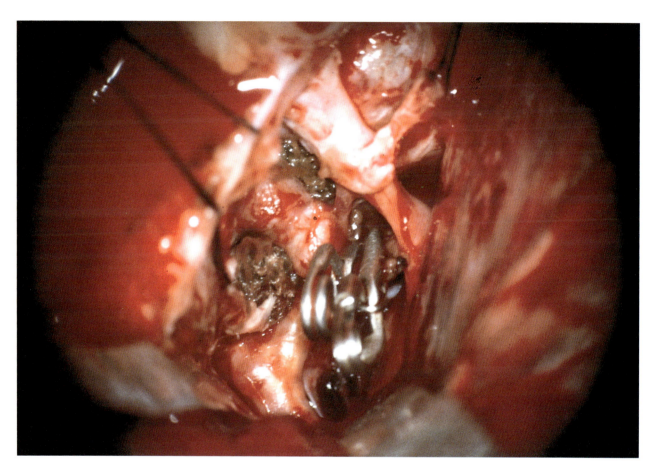

Fig. 90. The final situation after the application of the clips to the neck of the aneurysm is shown. The neck of the aneurysm peripherally from the clips is transected. The aneurysm sac is emptied and is left in place. Even if the aneurysm sac is completely or partially filled with blood clot or thrombus, the material from the inside of the sac should be removed and the sac left in situ. Removal of the sac itself is dangerous and most probably causes injury to the perforators for the hypothalamic area. The ON is no longer compressed. The clips are placed as far under and lateral to the ON as possible, so that they are not in contact with the nerve. The ophthalmic artery is completely dissected and its patency preserved. The extradural segment of the ICA in the anteromedial triangle is of normal diameter and so is the intradural segment of the ICA peripheral to the ophthalmic artery toward the posterior communicating artery (PCoA). The neck of the aneurysm is completely occluded. In the following step of the operation, watertight suturing of the dura is performed in the reverse order as when it was incised. In cases when it is not certain that the exposed mucous membrane of the ethmoid sinus and/or sphenoid sinus is intact, and if closure of the dura is not watertight, it is mandatory to seal all of those weak sites with pieces of muscle and fibrin glue in order to prevent a CSF leak. In all such cases where it is not completely certain that the dura has been watertightly sutured and when the bony sinuses were opened and sealed in order to prevent CSF leak, it is advisable that a lumbar drain be inserted for one week

SOF ICA (AL) DP (ON) ES OA

FL

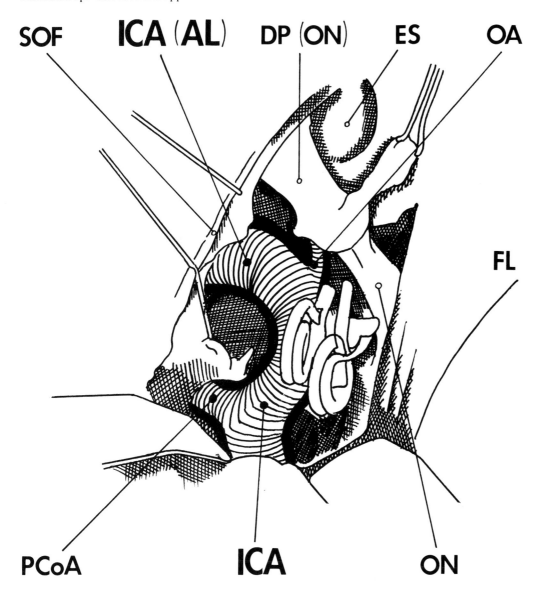

PCoA ICA ON

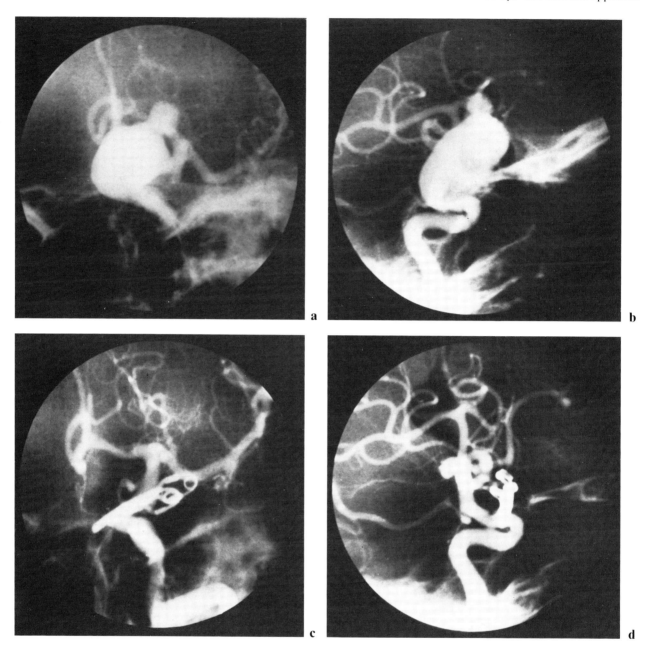

Fig. 91. Left carotid angiograms, anteroposterior views (**a, c**) and lateral views (**b, d**) of the same patient as presented in Figs. 83–90. **a, b** Preoperative angiograms showing a large carotid ophthalmic artery aneurysm. **c, d** Postoperative angiograms showing two clips on the carotid ophthalmic artery aneurysm. Both clips are placed more or less perpendicular over the ICA at the site of previously positioned aneurysm. Such placement of clips is far from ideal. The blades of the clips should be more along the longitudinal axis of the ICA. Filling of the ICA distal to the clips is satisfactory. The kinking of this segment seen intraoperatively in Fig. 89 does not show on the carotid angiogram on the lateral view (**d**)

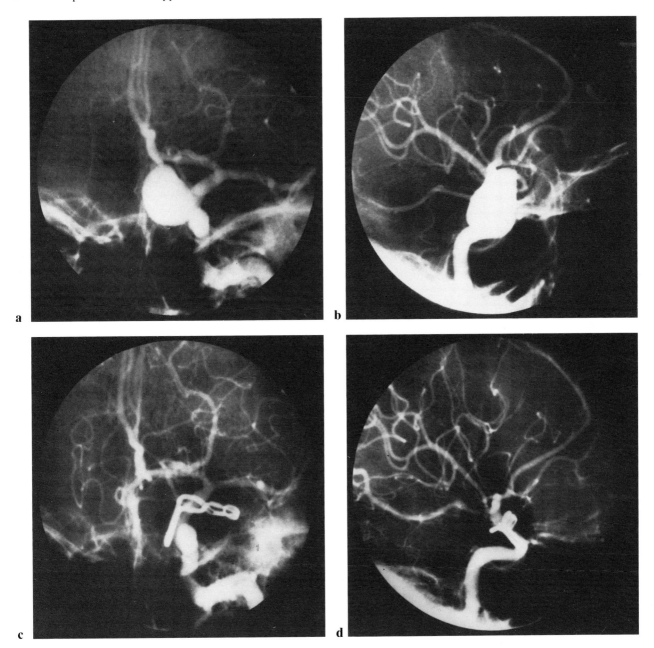

Fig. 92. Left carotid angiograms, anteroposterior views (**a, c**) and lateral views (**b, d**). **a, b** Preoperative angiograms showing a carotid ophthalmic artery aneurysm. **c, d** Postoperative angiograms showing a fenestrated clip on the carotid ophthalmic artery aneurysm. The ophthalmic artery can be seen proximal to the clip on the lateral view (**d**). The blades of the clip are properly positioned along the longitudinal axis of the ICA

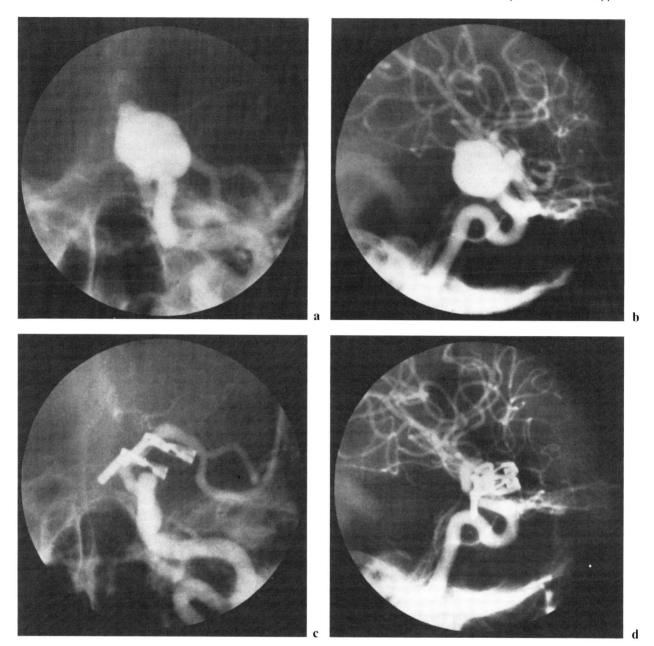

Fig. 93. Left carotid angiograms, anteroposterior views (**a, c**) and lateral views (**b, d**). **a, b** Preoperative angiograms showing a large carotid ophthalmic artery aneurysm. **c, d** Postoperative angiograms showing two fenestrated clips on the carotid ophthalmic artery aneurysm. Both clips are placed parallel in the same direction

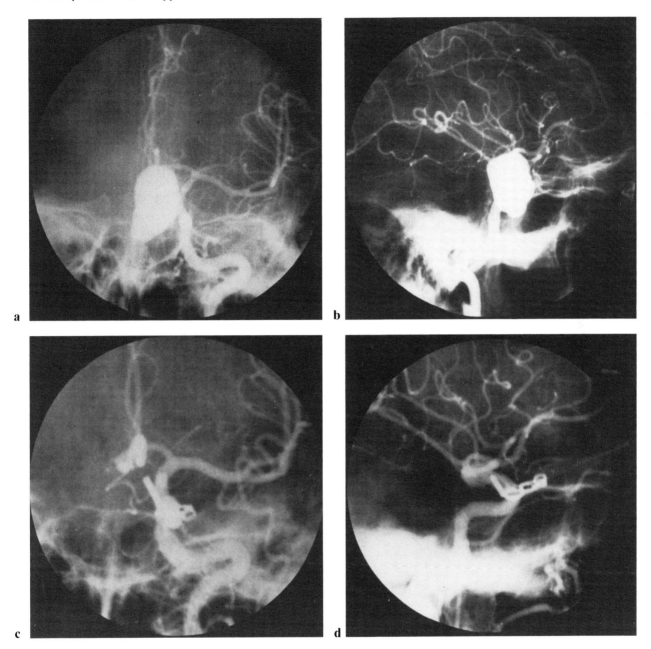

Fig. 94. Left carotid angiograms, anteroposterior views (**a, c**) and lateral views (**b, d**). **a, b** Preoperative angiograms showing a large carotid ophthalmic artery aneurysm. **c, d** Postoperative angiograms showing a fenestrated clip on the carotid ophthalmic artery aneurysm and normal arteries on the left side. The clip is properly placed along the longitudinal axis of the ICA

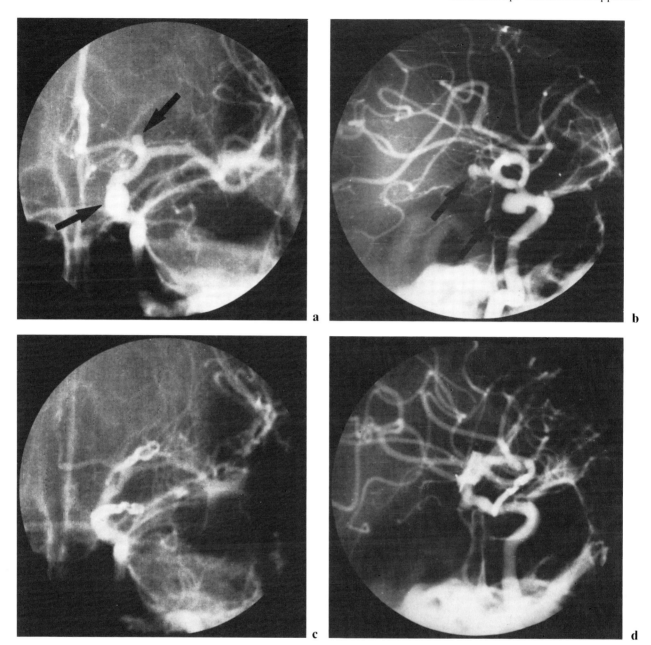

Fig. 95. Left carotid angiograms, anteroposterior views (**a, c**) and lateral views (**b, d**). **a, b** Preoperative angiograms showing two small aneurysms. The larger one is a carotid ophthalmic aneurysm, and the smaller is on the ICA at the bifurcation into the ACA and MCA. **c, d** Postoperative angiograms showing two clips, one on each aneurysm. The ophthalmic artery can be seen proximal to the clip on the lateral view (**d**)

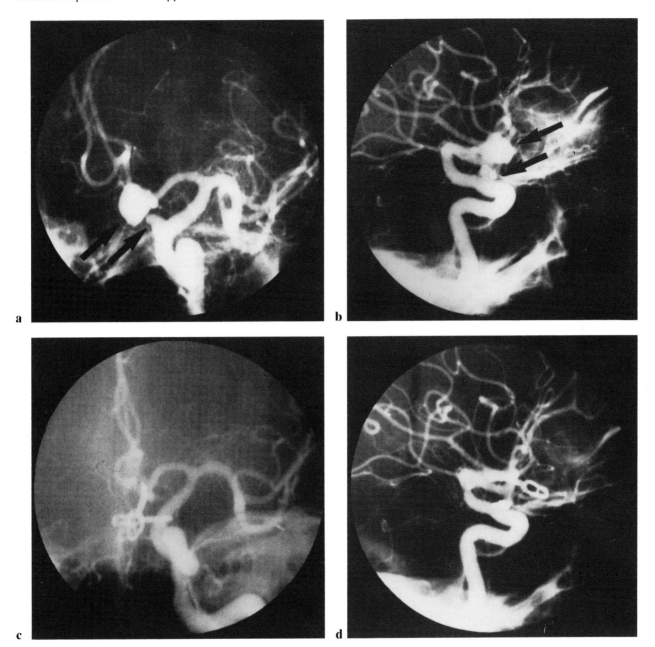

Fig. 96. Left carotid angiograms, anteroposterior views (**a, c**) and lateral views (**b, d**). **a, b** Preoperative angiograms showing a large ACoA aneurysm and a small carotid ophthalmic artery aneurysm. **c, d** Postoperative angiograms showing two clips, one on each aneurysm. The ophthalmic artery can be seen proximal to the clip on the lateral view (**d**)

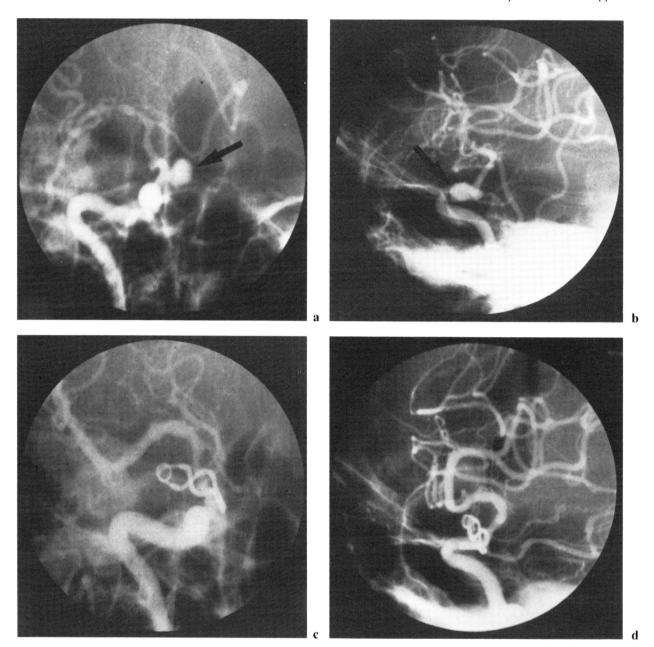

Fig. 97. Right carotid angiograms, anteroposterior views (**a, c**) and lateral views (**b, d**). **a, b** Preoperative angiograms showing a carotid ophthalmic artery aneurysm. **c, d** Postoperative angiograms showing a clip on the carotid ophthalmic artery aneurysm. The blades of the clip are properly positioned along the longitudinal axis of the ICA. The ophthalmic artery can be seen proximal to the clip on the lateral view (**d**)

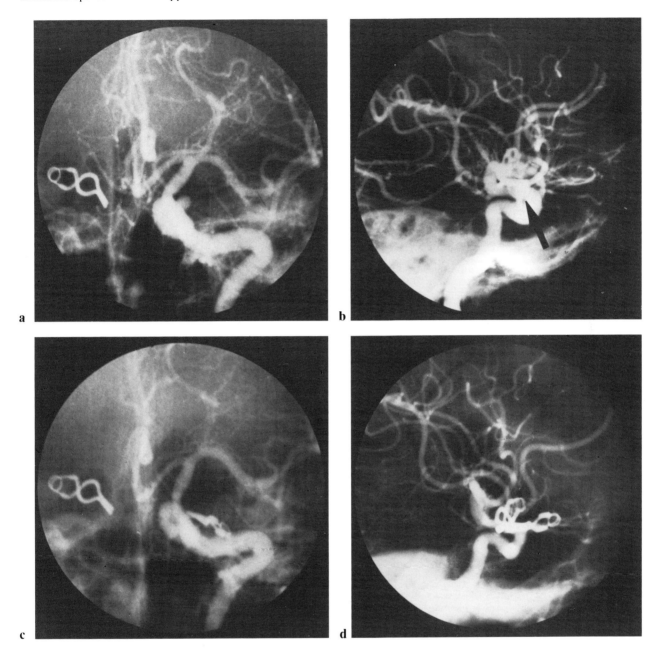

Fig. 98. Left carotid angiograms, anteroposterior views (**a, c**) and lateral views (**b, d**) of the same patient as shown in Fig. 97. **a, b** Postoperative angiograms of the first operation showing a fenestrated clip on the right side and a small aneurysm on the left carotid ophthalmic segment of the ICA. **c, d** Postoperative angiograms showing two clips, fenestrated on the right side and a nonfenestrated one on the left carotid ophthalmic aneurysm

3.2 Transclinoid-transcavernous-transsellar approach to basilar tip aneurysms

The idea for this approach arose for several reasons, the main being shortage of space at the time of placement of the clip on the aneurysm. Another important reason was insufficient visualization of the perforators situated behind the aneurysm due to the direction of the surgical approach used. According to the author's experience, shortage of space and insufficient visualization of perforators were found in most cases in which the aneurysm was larger than 1 cm in diameter, regardless of whether the approach used was pterional, lateral, or medial to the ICA or transsylvian, or subtemporal. Similar difficulties associated with a high risk of CSF leak were met in the transoral transclival approach to the distal basilar trunk and basilar tip aneurysms. The last, but not the least, important reason for a new approach to basilar tip aneurysms was the experience gained from dissection of fresh cadaver specimens of the sellar and parasellar region, as well as from a considerable number of operations in this area, among which the most important was surgery of carotid ophthalmic aneurysms, as well as surgery of tumorous lesions on the medial wall of the CS.

Using this approach, the basilar artery and aneurysm are approached from the ventral aspect which affords a good view of both sides of the basilar artery and the aneurysm. As this approach is a pterional one, it is clear that all the advantages of the original pterional approach, laterally as well as medially to the ICA, can be used. When this is not sufficient, however, the arachnoidea may be divided along the Sylvian fissure and the transsylvian approach used in addition. There is also a possibility of performing dissection of the IIIrd and IVth cranial nerves from the tentorial edge toward the SOF. In this way the IIIrd and IVth nerves can be moved medially and the tentorium incised posteriorly from the IVth nerve toward the Vth nerve, resulting in a large part of Parkinson's triangle being exposed and sufficient space being gained from the lateral side. By this maneuver, the basilar trunk is exposed in its upper half.

With the transclinoid-transcavernous-transsellar approach to the upper basilar trunk and basilar tip aneurysms, enough space is obtained for placement of the clip and for good visualization of all structures at the time of placement of the clip. Employing this approach, the basilar artery is always exposed enough proximally so that it is possible, whenever necessary, to place a temporary clip on it. What is especially important, is good bilateral visualization from the ventral aspect of both sides of the basilar artery and the aneurysm, enabling identification of the perforating vessels, which are, in the case of large and giant aneurysms of the basilar tip, displaced to both sides, and usually tightly adherent to the aneurysm itself.

The transclinoid-transcavernous-transsellar approach does not exclude any of the previous approaches; on the contrary, it does or at least it may further increase the advantage which any one of the standard approaches offers when used in combination. The controversy surrounding this allegedly dangerous approach can only be overcome by experimental microanatomical dissections of cadaver specimens prior to reaching a decision to practice this approach on patients with this type of aneurysm.

The initial placement and fixation of the patient's head is the same as in operations for carotid ophthalmic aneurysms [57], i.e., position 1 shown in Fig. 67. It goes without saying that in surgery for left carotid opthalmic aneurysms the patient's head will be turned to the right and vice versa. However, it is necessary to point out that, as the basilar tip aneurysms are mostly situated in the sagittal plane, the approach of the right-handed neurosurgeon will be from the right, and only exceptionally from the left side, if the position of the aneurysm dictates it. For a left-handed surgeon, a more convenient approach will be from the left side, again if the position and the projection of the aneurysm do not require the opposite. The skin incision, the craniotomy, and the dural opening are made in the same way and in the same extent as in operations for carotid ophthalmic aneurysms. The procedure for the unroofing of the optic canal, as well as for the complete removal of the ACP, is also the same. Special attention should be paid to the possibility of accidental opening of the frontal, ethmoid, and/or sphenoid bony sinuses, and to possible injury to the mucous membrane of these sinuses. In this event, the watertight closure of such an aperture must be performed. Of paramount importance in surgery of both carotid ophthalmic aneurysms and basilar tip aneurysms is the preservation of normal intradural volume and pressure of the CSF during craniotomy and throughout the epidural stage of the operation. Care must be taken not to damage the dura, and to prevent a CSF leak. Lumbar drainage and removal of the CSF must not be performed before the epidural step of the operation is completed and the dura is opened. The incision of the dura is identical as in surgery for carotid ophthalmic aneurysms and is shown in Figs. 84–88. The temporal and frontal lobes are gently retracted to expose the intradural portion of the ICA, its bifurcation into the MCA and ACA as well as all the branches running from the ACA and from the site of the bifurcation of the ICA (Fig. 100).

Subsequently in the procedure, the intradural segment of the ON, the initial part of the optic tract, the IIIrd nerve and the PCP are exposed (Figs. 100 and 101). Even though in some cases the slit between the ON and the ACA appears larger than the slit between the ICA and the IIIrd nerve (Fig. 100), the procedure should be performed in the area between the ICA and the IIIrd nerve (Fig. 101). Reason for this decision is that despite the fact that at the beginning the operative area between the ICA and the IIIrd nerve may be smaller than on the medial aspect of the ICA toward the ON and the ACA, the space between the ICA and the IIIrd nerve can be enlarged at least by a factor of 3 so that the anteromedial triangle posterior to the anterior loop of the ICA in the CS and in the sella is used (Figs. 102–105). The space between the ICA, the ON and the ACA, however, is restricted and cannot be enlarged by retraction of any of those three structures without high probability of damage to them (Fig. 100).

The incision into the dura propria over the ON is made along the longitudinal axis of the ON in the optic canal. In this way, the ON is exposed and on its inferior and lateral aspect the ophthalmic artery is visualized running along the ON (Fig. 4). The dural ring is cut circumferentially around the ICA, thus enabling the displacement of the ICA medially together with the ophthalmic artery and the ON. The enlargement of the anteromedial triangle could be achieved also toward the lateral side by dissection of the IIIrd nerve from its entry point to the lateral wall of the CS toward the SOF (Fig. 5). The IIIrd nerve is dissected and displaced laterally (Fig. 102). Then the diaphragm of the sella is cut in transverse direction in front of the PCP and dorsum sellae to the midline where the pituitary stalk enters

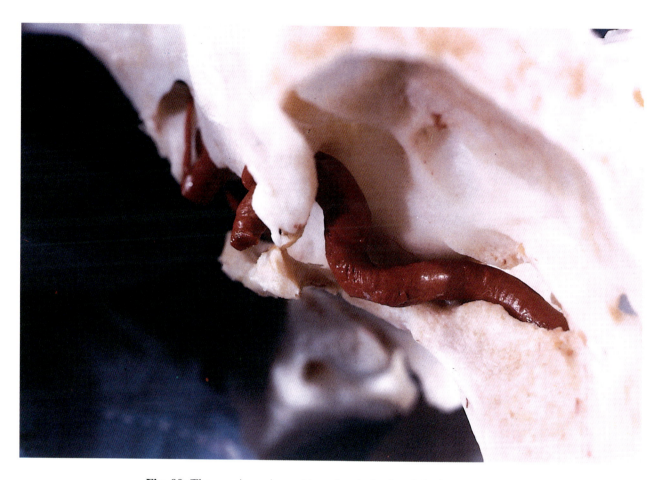

Fig. 99. The specimen is positioned as is the head during surgery while removing the ACP and PCP, i.e., position 3 (Fig. 67). The anterior loop of the ICA is almost in the horizontal plane. Following complete resection of the sphenoid wing, the ACP and PCP, sufficient space is gained posterior to the anterior loop of the ICA through the CS and sella onto the posterior cranial fossa so that the upper segment of the basilar artery with its bifurcation is easily reached

the diaphragm of the sella. Surgicel is placed in front of the PCP into the sella to stop bleeding from the posterior intercavernous sinus. Surgicel is also placed on the lateral aspect of the PCP onto the CS, on the medial aspect of the horizontal segment of the ICA, and on the medial aspect of the medial loop of the ICA. The anterior-intrasellar aspect of the PCP is exposed from the tip of the PCP to the very bottom of the sella (Fig. 102). Anteriorly in the sella the pituitary body is

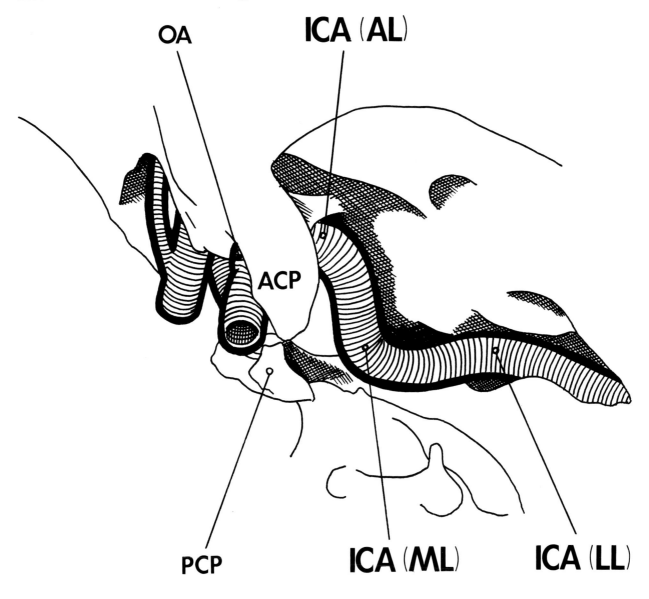

OA ICA (AL)

ACP

PCP ICA (ML) ICA (LL)

visualized on its lateral and dorsal aspects (Fig. 102). The drilling of the PCP is commenced from the intrasellar direction backwards. The PCP is drilled off completely down to the bottom of the sella and the dura overlying the PCP on its posterior aspect is pushed forward or excised (Figs. 103 and 104). The PCP with its base and overlying dura are excised far enough down so that a sufficient view of the neck of the aneurysm is obtained. The upper segment of the basilar artery is

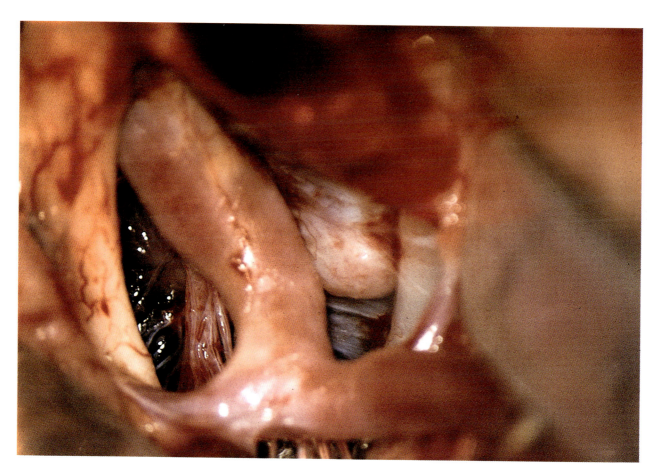

Fig. 100. Intraoperative view of the compartments between the ON and ICA and between the ICA and the IIIrd nerve. Through the slit between the ICA and the ON several perforating arteries are shown. Because these arteries are of vital importance to the ON, optic chiasm and optic tract, pituitary stalk, and hypothalamus, they should be preserved at all cost during surgery. Displacement of the ICA laterally would cause stretching of these arteries resulting in vasospasm and possible thrombosis. On the lateral side of the ICA the PCP, Lilieqvist membrane, and the IIIrd nerve can be seen. Displacement of the ICA medially does not endanger the perforators arising from the ICA on its inferomedial aspect

exposed thus providing enough space for placement of a temporary clip on the basilar artery, if necessary, for safe dissection of the aneurysm and perforators, and finally safe and proper placement of a definitive clip on the neck of the aneurysm (Figs. 104 and 105).

Figures 99–105 show the transclinoid-transcavernous-transsellar approach from the right side to the basilar tip and the upper basilar trunk.

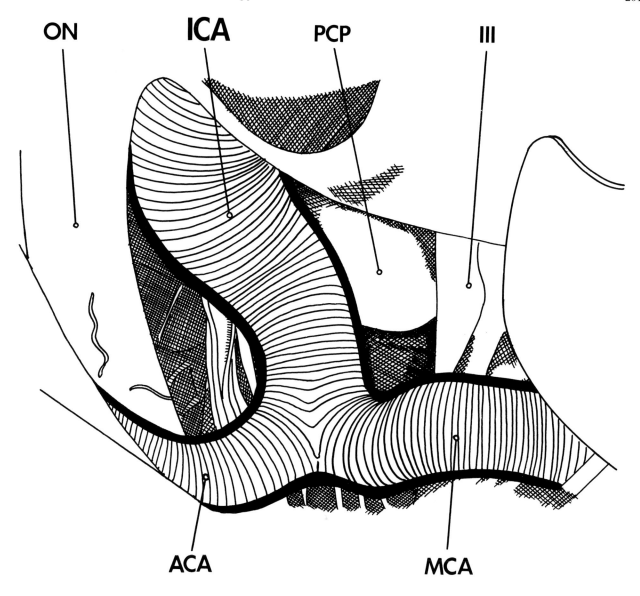

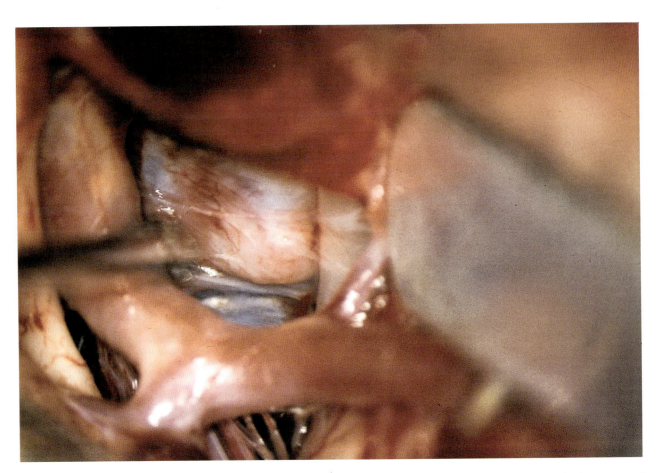

Fig. 101. Intraoperative view of the PCP with the ICA displaced medially. Displacement of the ICA medially does not affect the function of the perforators running from the inferomedial aspect of the ICA, nor the ophthalmic artery, ON, optic chiasm, ACA, MCA, and perforators running from the under aspect of the bifurcation of the ICA into the ACA, and MCA. The IIIrd nerve on the lateral aspect of the PCP is also not affected by displacement of the ICA. Note: retraction of the ICA should be very gentle and "dynamic". To put a fixed spatula over the ICA might be dangerous and could produce vasospasm of the artery wall. To avoid this, short-lasting gentle retraction performed by a suction tube is the only way to preserve the integrity and normal function of the ICA

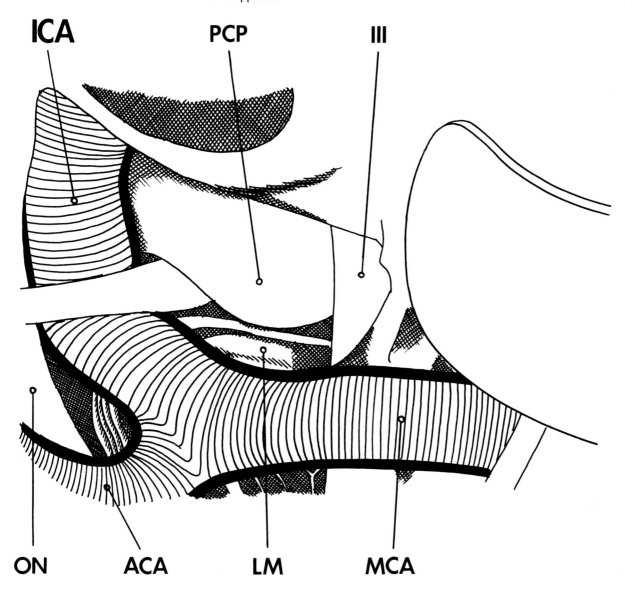

ICA   **PCP**   **III**

ON   **ACA**   **LM**   **MCA**

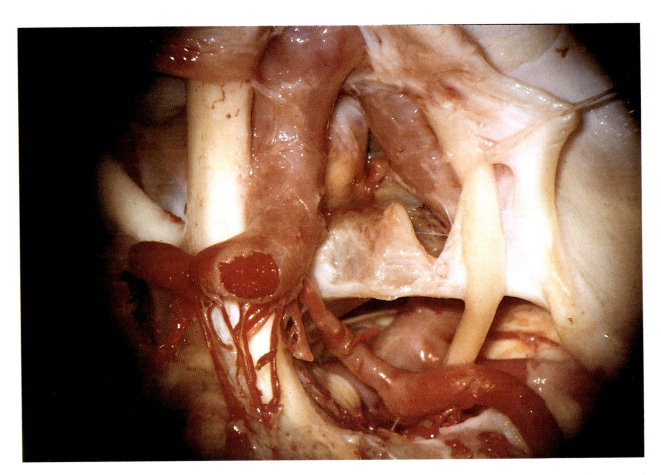

Fig. 102. A fresh cadaver specimen with arterial injection showing the relationships around the PCP, which is still in situ. The diaphragm of the sella, the dura over the apex of the PCP and distal dural ring around the ICA have been removed. The horizontal segment of the intracavernous ICA, the concave side of the anterior loop of the ICA and the medial aspect of the medial loop of the ICA are shown in the CS. The pituitary body and the artery running from the MHT to the pituitary body are shown in the sella. The anteromedial triangle has been opened and the edge of the tentorium fixed with a suture and pulled laterally, providing lateral displacement of the IIIrd nerve thus allowing access to the lateral side of the PCP. Posterior to the PCP the basilar artery bifurcation, right SCA, right PCA and PCoA are shown. Note: The area behind the PCP medial to the IIIrd nerve and lateral to the PCoA is much smaller than the area delineated by the concave side of the anterior loop of the ICA anteriorly, by the lateral aspect of the intradural ICA medially, by the medial aspect of the horizontal segment of the intracavernous ICA and by the posterior margin of the PCP. It is obvious that the PCP is the main obstacle to the upper segment of the basilar artery as indicated by the arrow

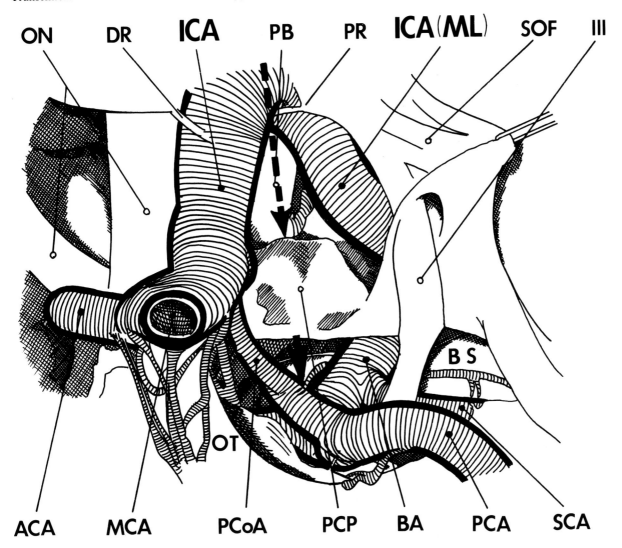

ON DR **ICA** PB PR **ICA(ML)** SOF III

B S

OT

ACA MCA PCoA PCP BA PCA SCA

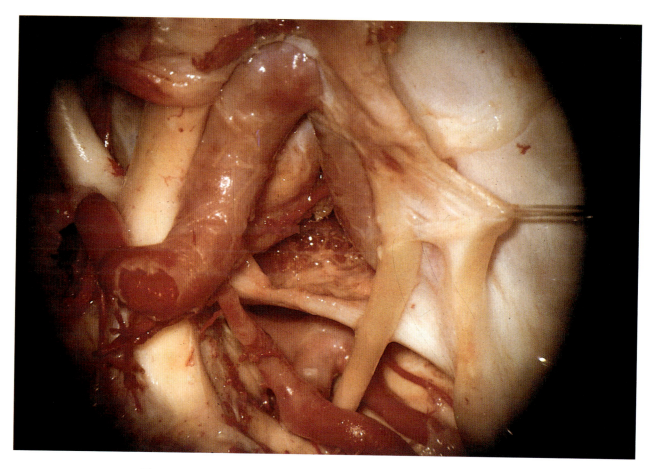

Fig. 103. The PCP has been completely resected. The dura overlying the posterior aspect of the PCP is still in situ. The pituitary body with the capsular artery in the sella, the posterior aspect of the anterior loop and the medial aspect of the horizontal loop of the ICA in the CS, are shown. Bifurcation of the basilar artery to both PCAs is seen in the depth underneath the dura of the posterior side of the PCP. It is obvious that the approach to the bifurcation of the basilar artery and to its upper segment is hampered by the dura covering the posterior side of the PCP which is still in place, as indicated by the arrow

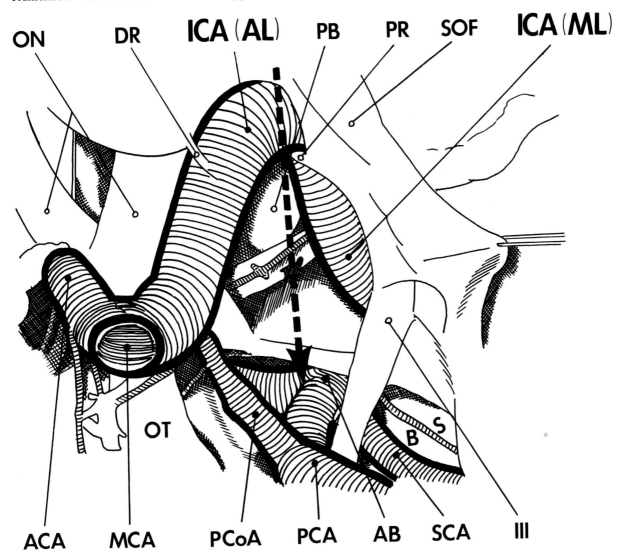

ON DR ICA (AL) PB PR SOF ICA (ML)

OT

B S

ACA MCA PCoA PCA AB SCA III

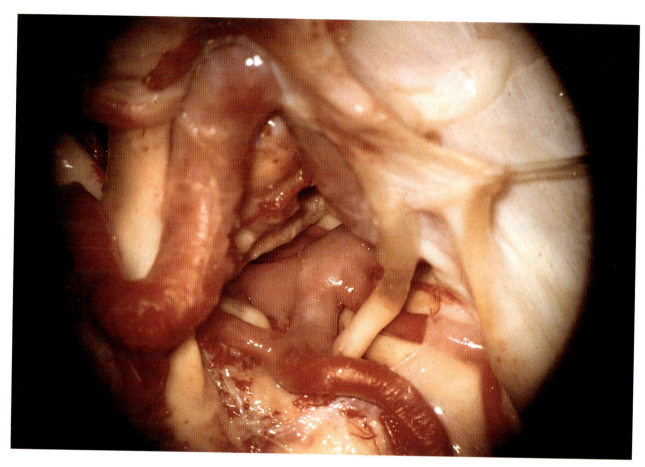

Fig. 104. The dura of the posterior side of the PCP has been resected. With the complete removal of the PCP and resection of the dura overlying the posterior aspect of the PCP, the "corridor" toward the upper part of the basilar artery with its bifurcation has been sufficiently enlarged. Bifurcation of the basilar artery, both PCAs, both SCAs, right PCoA, the IIIrd nerve, intracavernous and intradural ICA, and the pituitary body are sufficiently visualized and can be fully preserved during surgery for the basilar tip aneurysm

ON   DR   **ICA (AL)**   PR   SOF   PB   **ICA(ML)**

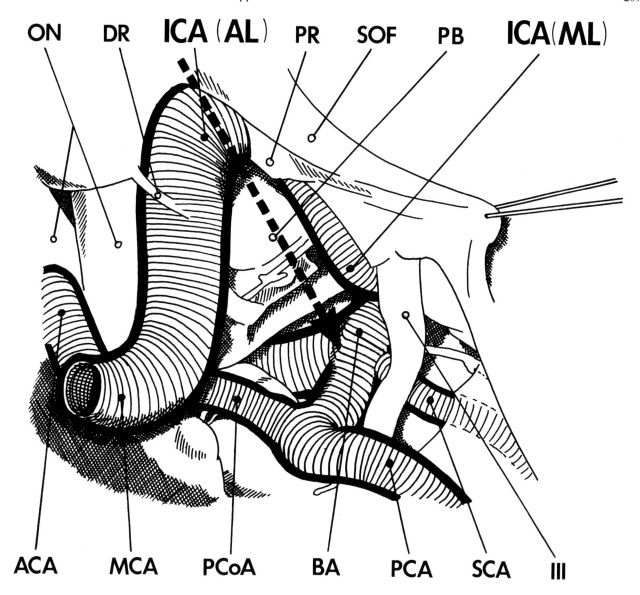

ACA   MCA   PCoA   BA   PCA   SCA   III

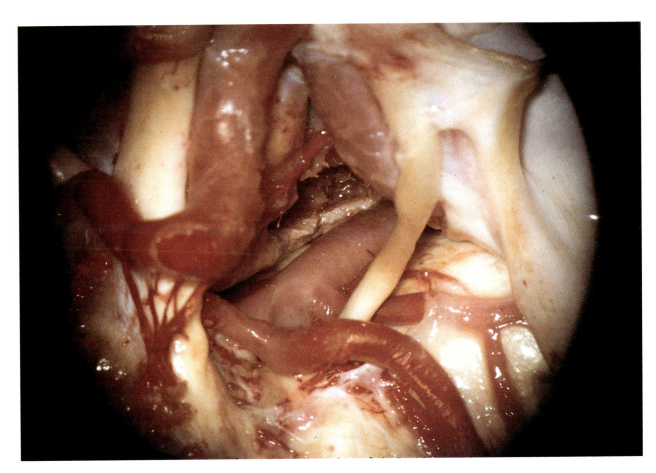

Fig. 105. In cases of large and giant basilar tip aneurysms, sufficient exposure of the proximal segment of the basilar artery is mandatory. For this reason, additional resection of the base of the PCP or even part of the clivus should be undertaken, and the dura overlying the bony structures excised. Extensive resection of the bone and the overlying dura, together with the change in position of the head (Fig. 67) from position 3 to position 1 or even to position 2, as in this figure, allows sufficient access to the basilary trunk and placement of a temporary clip on the basilar artery, when necessary. By appropriate exposure of the basilar artery and its bifurcation only slight, if any, retraction of the brain, is necessary

ON   DR   ICA   PB   PR SOF ICA(ML) BA

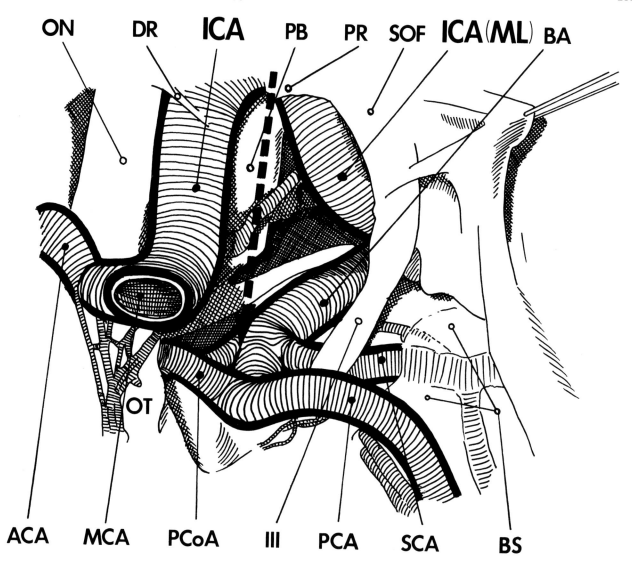

ACA   MCA   PCoA   III   PCA   SCA   BS

OT

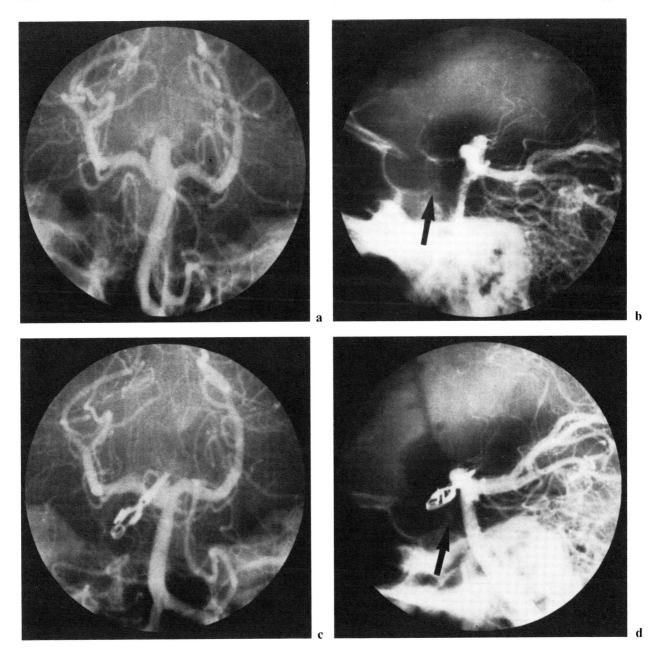

Fig. 106. Vertebral angiograms, anteroposterior views (**a, c**) and lateral views (**b, d**). **a, b** Preoperative angiograms showing a small irregular and eccentric basilar tip aneurysm positioned to the right side. **c, d** Postoperative angiograms showing a clip on the neck of the basilar tip aneurysm at the origin of the posterior cerebral artery from the bifurcation of the basilar artery on the right side. **b, d** The arrow points to the portion of the PCP which was drilled off on the right side

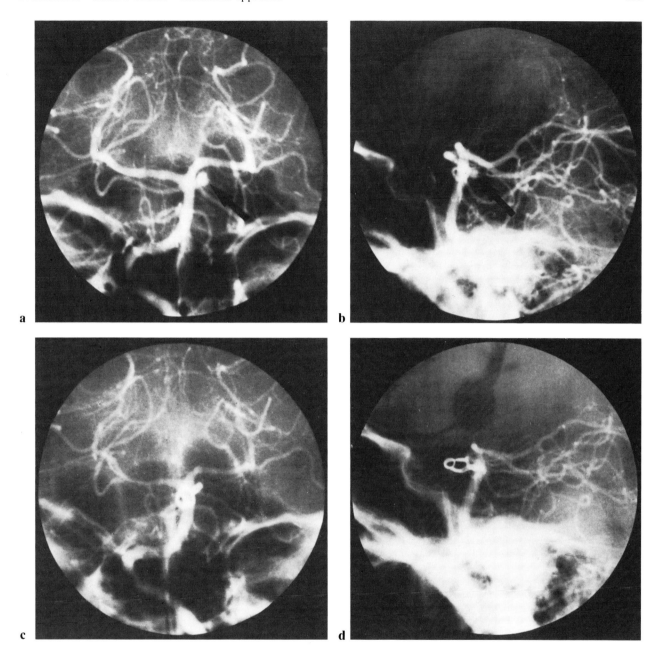

Fig. 107. Vertebral angiograms, anteroposterior views (**a, c**) and lateral views (**b, d**) **a, b** Preoperative angiograms showing a small aneurysm on the left side of the basilar artery between the superior cerebellar artery and posterior cerebral artery. **b** The arrow points to the aneurysm and the irregular shape of the fundus where it ruptured. **c, d** Postoperative angiograms showing a clip on the left side of the basilar artery between the superior cerebellar artery and posterior cerebral artery. The aneurysm is completely occluded

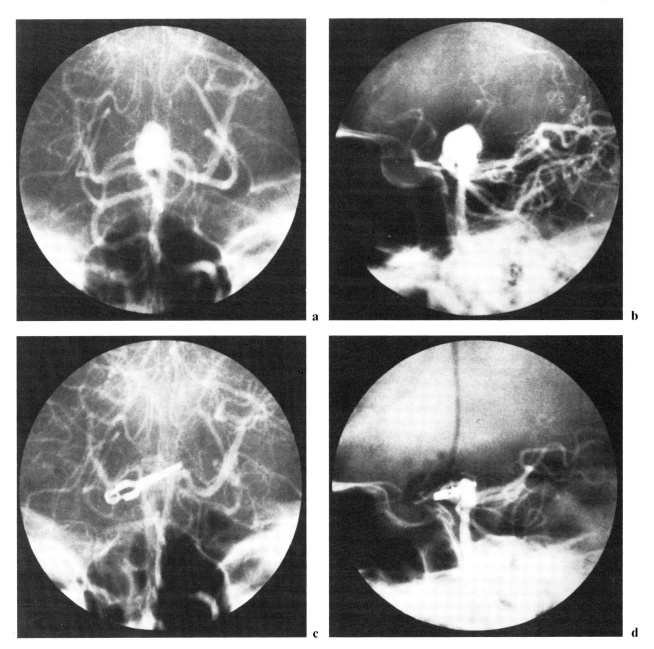

Fig. 108. Vertebral angiograms, anteroposterior views (**a, c**) and lateral views (**b, d**). **a, b** Preoperative angiograms showing an irregular basilar tip aneurysm. **c, d** Postoperative angiograms showing a clip on the basilar tip and no aneurysm. Note that the basilar tip is a little lower than the tip of the PCP and close to it

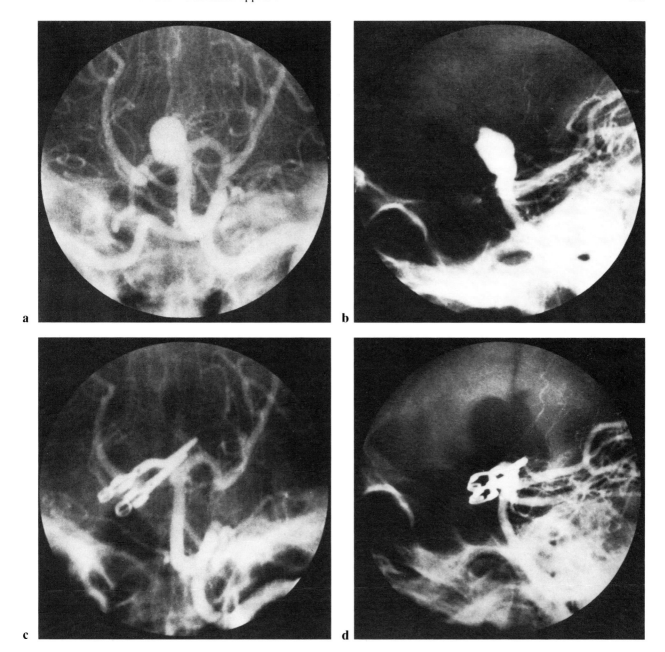

Fig. 109. Vertebral angiograms, anteroposterior views (**a, c**) and lateral views (**b, d**). **a, b** Preoperative angiograms showing a medium-sized irregular basilar tip aneurysm projecting upwards and frontwards. **c, d** Postoperative angiograms showing two clips on the basilar tip, no aneurysm, and normal bifurcation of the basilar artery

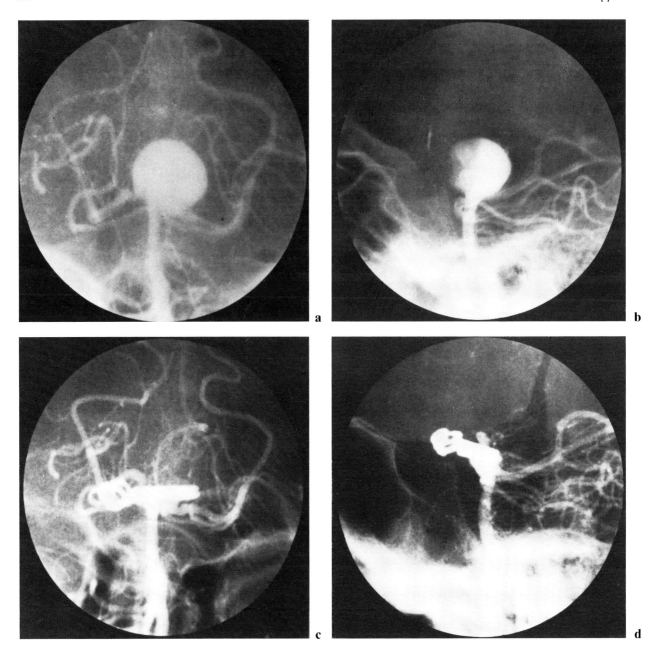

Fig. 110. Vertebral angiograms, anteroposterior views (**a, c**) and lateral views (**b, d**). **a, b** Preoperative angiograms showing a large basilar tip aneurysm. **c, d** Postoperative angiograms showing two clips on the basilar tip. The aneurysm is completely occluded. Note the irregular shape and density of the anterior half of the aneurysm which is due to the turbulence of the stream of dye (**b**)

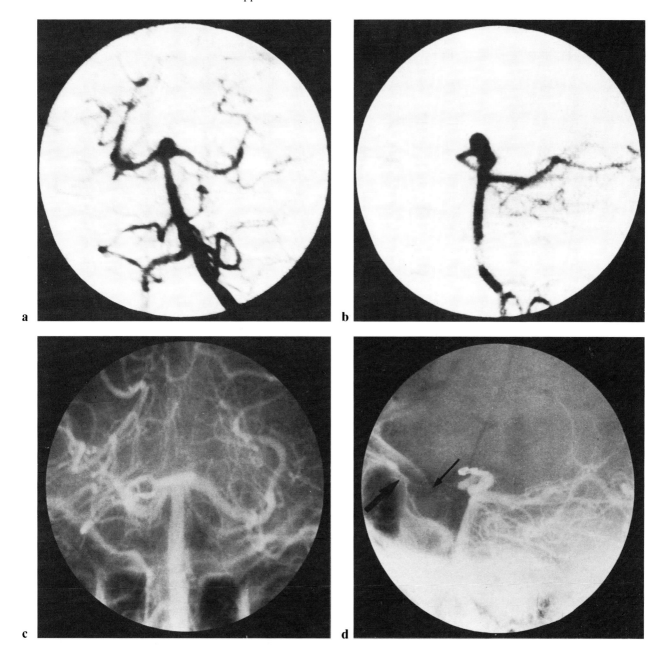

Fig. 111. Vertebral angiograms, anteroposterior views (**a, c**) and lateral views (**b, d**). **a, b** Preoperative angiograms showing a small basilar tip aneurysm. **c, d** Postoperative angiograms showing a clip on the basilar tip. The aneurysm is excluded and the bifurcation of the basilar artery is of normal configuration. **d** The thicker arrow indicates the base of the resected ACP while the thinner arrow points to the normal ACP on the left side

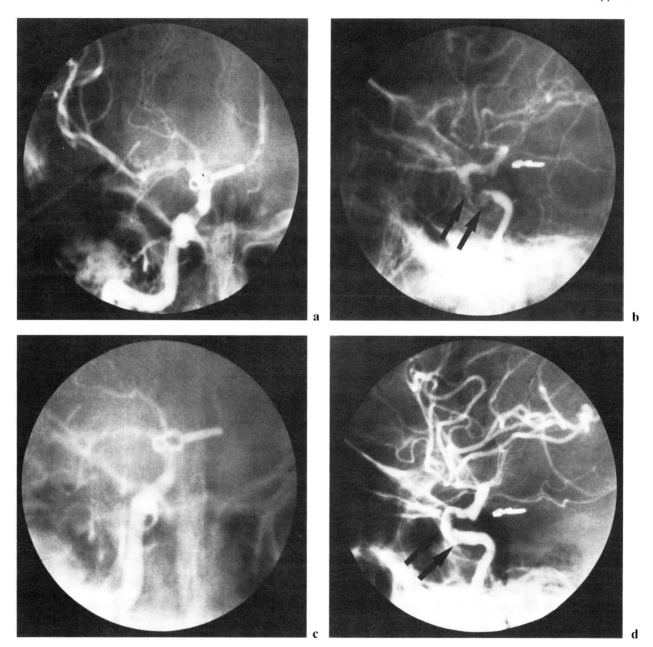

Fig. 112. Right carotid angiograms of the same patient as presented in Fig. 111, anteroposterior views (**a, c**) and lateral views (**b, d**). **a, b** Preoperative angiograms following the initial surgery for a basilar tip aneurysm showing the filling defect on the horizontal segment and on the anterior loop of the ICA in the CS. **c, d** Postoperative angiograms showing almost normal filling of the intracavernous portion of the ICA. **b, d** Arrows pointing to the length of the filling defect. The clip is on the tip of the basilar artery. The stenosis and filling defect of the ICA in the CS were caused by too much Surgicel having been placed on the lateral aspect of the PCP during the initial operation (**a, b**). At the second operation, Surgicel was partially removed and better filling of the ICA in the CS was achieved (**c, d**)

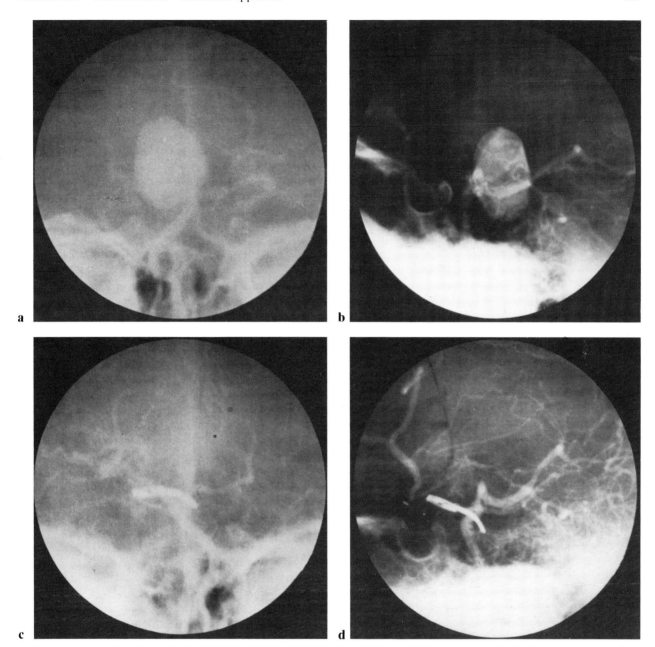

Fig. 113. Vertebral angiograms, anteroposterior views (**a, c**) and lateral views (**b, d**). **a, b** Preoperative angiograms showing a large basilar tip aneurysm projecting slightly to the right side. **c, d** Postoperative angiograms showing a Yasargil clip on the basilar tip. The aneurysm is excluded, and the configuration of the basilar artery is preserved intact

4.1 Intracavernous (saccular, fusiform) aneurysms of the internal carotid artery

Intracavernous saccular and fusiform aneurysms of the ICA can be located anywhere from the lateral to the distal dural rings of the ICA. Most of them are located on the concave aspect of the anterior loop of the intracavernous ICA. The intracavernous aneurysms vary not only in location but also in size. Symptoms and signs of local compression of the surrounding structures only occur when the aneurysm is large or giant. However, small intracavernous aneurysms may be responsible for TIA due to aneurysm to artery embolism. This is much more true for large and giant intracavernous aneurysms which are partially thrombosed or filled with blood clot. Small intracavernous aneurysms may rupture and cause CCFs. Large and giant aneurysms of the ICA in the CS are the origin of emboli to the peripheral cerebral vascular tree in a much higher proportion than small intracavernous ICA aneurysms. At the same time, large and giant ICA intracavernous aneurysms cause local symptoms, due to compression of the surrounding structures thus causing paresis of nerves III through VI. Headache caused by large and/or giant intracavernous aneurysms is usually more disturbing than headache caused by tumorous lesions of the CS. While rupture of a small intracavernous aneurysm usually leads to a CCF and only occasionally to a large or giant false aneurysm, rupture of a large or giant aneurysm is much more dangerous and may, along with the local symptoms and signs, also cause intradural catastrophic hemorrhage [14]. Small intracavernous aneurysms in most cases are discovered incidentally during carotid angiography in patients with SAH, due to the rupture of an aneurysm intradurally. Large and giant aneurysms of the ICA in the CS are, in most cases, diagnosed by CT scan performed because of headache. The diagnosis in such cases is then confirmed by carotid angiography on the side of the lesion in the CS. When direct surgical approach is planned for a small, large, or giant intracavernous aneurysm, four vessel angiography should be performed together with cross studies.

The ideal treatment of any aneurysm is the complete exclusion of the lesion from the circulation, with the preservation of the patency of the artery from which the aneurysm grew. The same is true for intracavernous ICA aneurysms. When the intracavernous ICA aneurysm can be excluded, reduced in size and the patency of the ICA preserved by the detachable balloon technique, it is self-evident that a direct surgical approach is not necessary. However, in many intracavernous ICA aneurysms the defect in the vessel wall is too large, and the balloon can easily drop into the lumen of the artery and compromise its patency. If this is the case, the direct surgical approach is preferable and reconstruction of the arterial wall after the exclusion of the aneurysm is attempted. The exclusion of the aneurysm is possible by clipping or excision. When the intracavernous aneurysm has to be resected, the wall of the artery should be repaired by interrupted sutures and/or by clipping.

Whenever resection of the aneurysm is performed, temporary exclusion of the whole intracavernous segment of the ICA from the circulation is necessary. Temporary clips are put on the posterior loop of the ICA through the posterolateral triangle (Figs. 26–30) and on the anterior loop of the ICA in the anteromedial triangle (Figs. 1–3). Resection of the aneurysm and reconstruction of the ICA wall by suturing or clipping or both should be completed in half an hour, even if the cross circulation has been proven satisfactory. If the defect of the artery wall is too extensive and the wall of the aneurysm too weak, and direct reconstruction is impossible, the saphenous vein is used for a graft which is interposed between the posterior and the anterior loops of the ICA.

Most small intracavernous ICA aneurysms located on the anterior loop or horizontal segment of the ICA between the medial and the anterior loop can be reached through the anteromedial and/or paramedial triangle (Figs. 1–10). When an aneurysm is located on the medial loop of the ICA or even more proximally toward the lateral ring of the ICA, an approach through Parkinson's triangle is necessary (Figs. 11–14).

In most cases of large and/or giant aneurysms, the anterior loop of the ICA is dissected in the anteromedial triangle. Dissection of the ICA then proceeds proximally along the horizontal segment of the ICA from its anterior loop toward its medial loop until the neck of the aneurysm is reached. If it is necessary, the IIIrd and the IVth nerves are dissected along their course in the lateral wall of the CS toward the orbit. In this way, first, the anteromedial triangle may be enlarged and if this is not enough, the paramedial triangle may be opened and enlarged, and, finally, Parkinson's triangle is opened. When the aneurysm is reached in cases of large and giant aneurysms and if the neck is wide, the circulation through the intracavernous segment of the ICA is temporarily excluded by placing clips on the posterior and anterior loops of the ICA. The sac of the aneurysm is then incised and the aneurysm entered. The defect of the ICA wall is checked after removal of the blood clot or thrombus from the aneurysm, if there is any.

In most large and giant aneurysms, unless they are fusiform, reconstruction of the ICA wall is possible by clipping and/or by suturing. Only when there is fusiform dilatation of the ICA, is by-pass vein grafting usually necessary.

In many large and/or giant ICA intracavernous aneurysms, it is impossible to be sure before inspecting the interior of the aneurysm which type of reconstruction of the ICA will be necessary. Whenever the possibility exists that grafting of the artery may be needed, the saphenous vein should be prepared in advance.

In surgery of large and giant intracavernous aneurysms, there is almost no venous bleeding because the CS no longer exists. However, in cases of small intracavernous aneurysms, the major part of the CS still functions and venous bleeding might be a problem. Surgicel is packed around the ICA step-wise from the anterior loop of the ICA proximally towards the aneurysm. When the aneurysm is isolated and clipped, Surgicel is removed and the whole space around the aneurysm and around the ICA is checked to ensure that there is not too much Surgicel and that the diameter of the ICA is normal. At the end of the operation, only a small amount of Surgicel is packed into the CS around the ICA completely stopping venous bleeding.

While in most small intracavernous ICA aneurysms the best clip is the ring clip which embraces the aneurysm together with the artery, care should be taken that the part of the clip which projects away from both the aneurysm and the artery, and which is more bulky than the usual clip, does not compress any of the nerves II through VI.

In cases of large and giant aneurysms when the neck of the aneurysm is transsected, the ICA wall is reconstructed, and the blood clot or thrombus from the aneurysm sac is removed, the sac of the aneurysm is left in place so as not to damage the nerves. Care must be taken particularly of the VIth nerve, which in most cases is stretched far laterally and posteriorly over the aneurysmal sac. Whenever reconstruction of the ICA by suturing, clipping, or grafting after resection of the aneurysm takes a longer period of time, and in cases where cross circulation is poor, barbiturate protection of the brain is advisable.

Consecutive stages of the surgery for a left sided intracavernous ICA aneurysm are presented in Figs. 115–121. Figure 114 shows an asymptomatic aneurysm which was found at the dissection of the CS and represents an "incidental" finding during autopsy.

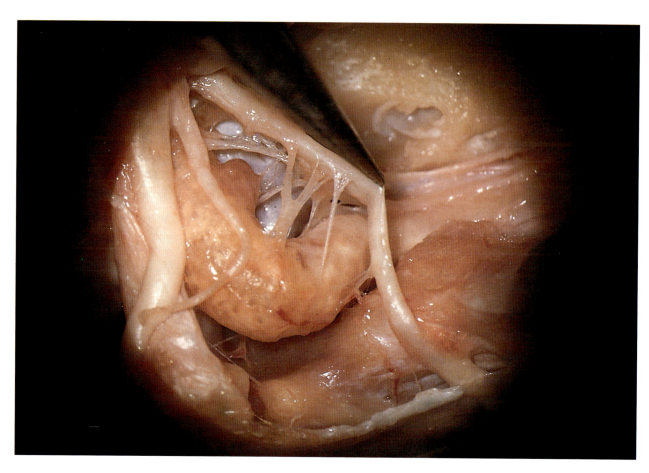

Fig. 114. A small intracavernous ICA aneurysm is situated on the horizontal segment of the ICA and projects inferolaterally. A number of sympathetic fibers running from the ICA to the VIth nerve, and the VIth nerve itself, are stretched over the dome of the aneurysm. The IIIrd and the IVth nerves are shown. The Vth nerve with the GG has been removed. The lateral and medial loops of the ICA are visualized. The MHT is seen on the medial aspect of the medial loop of the ICA

A   SNN

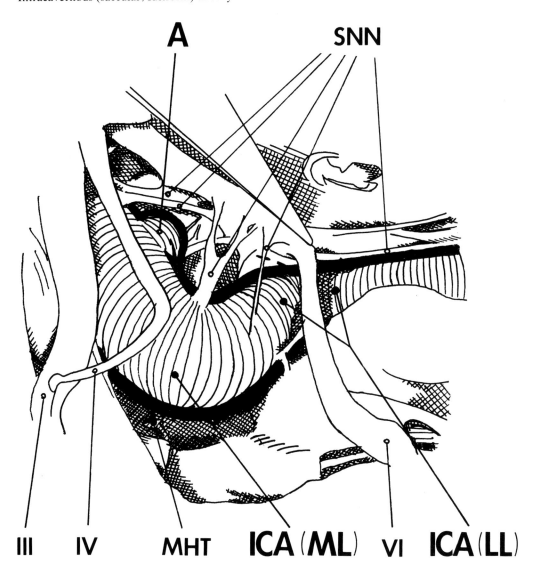

III   IV   MHT   **ICA(ML)**   VI   **ICA(LL)**

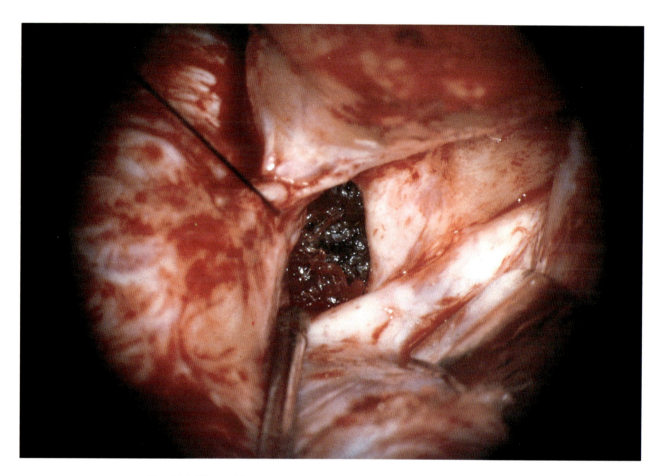

Fig. 115. The epidural stage of the direct surgical approach to the intracavernous aneurysm of the left ICA has been completed. The orbital roof, the sphenoid wing with the ACP, and the walls of the optic canal have been removed. The lateral tip of the SOF has been fixed with a stay suture. The anteromedial triangle is presented epidurally. The ON has been explored in its entire length in the optic canal and is still covered by the dura propria

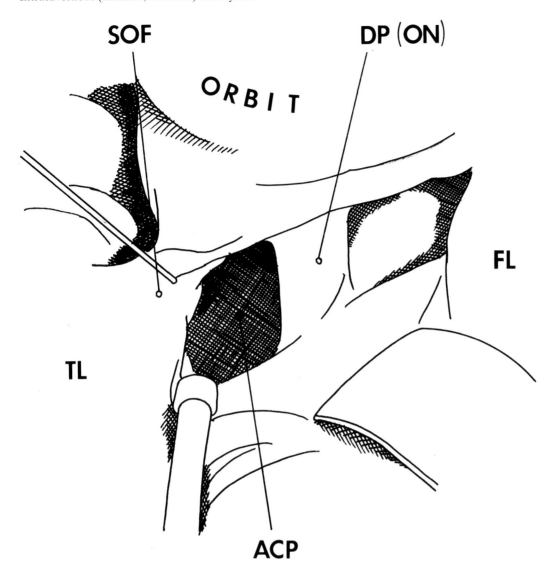

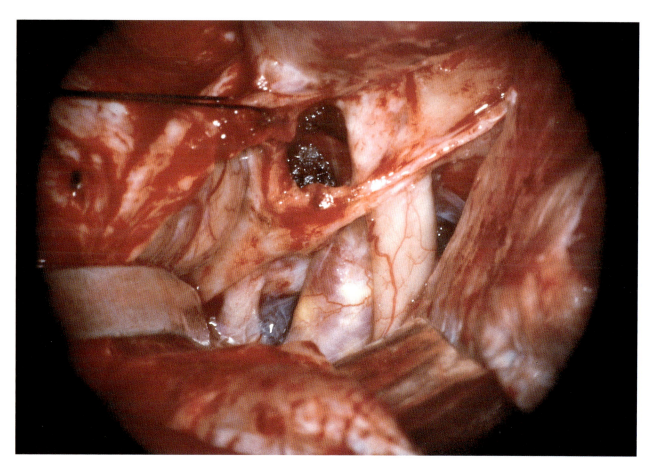

Fig. 116. The dura has been opened on the medial aspect of the SOF and transversely over the IIIrd nerve, the ICA and the ON. The ON can be seen both intradurally and extradurally in its entire length in the optic canal. The ICA is shown intradurally on the lateral aspect of the ON and extradurally in the anteromedial triangle, where the anterior loop of the ICA can be traced. More laterally, the IIIrd nerve can be seen intradurally and at the site of entry to the lateral wall of the CS forming the lateral border of the anteromedial triangle. Intradurally between the ICA and the IIIrd nerve the PCP is seen

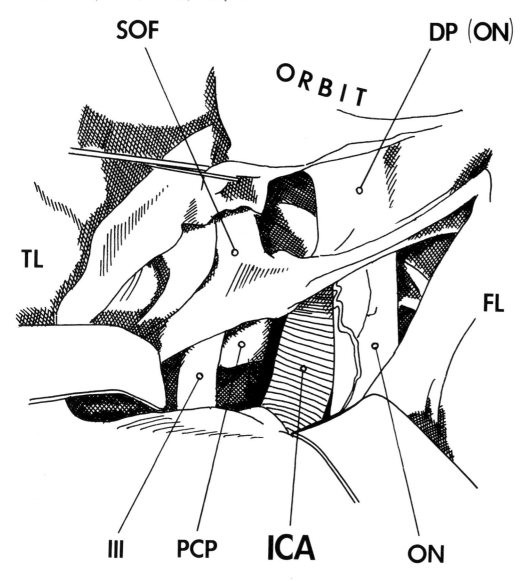

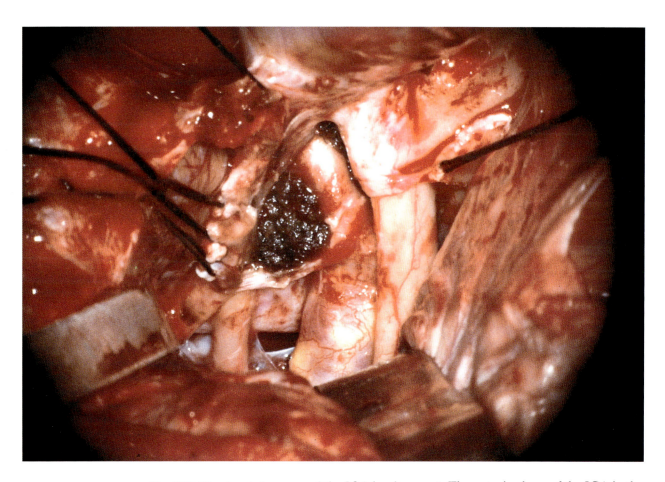

Fig. 117. The dural ring around the ICA has been cut. The anterior loop of the ICA in the anteromedial triangle is exposed. The proximal ring of the ICA in the anteromedial triangle is still in place. Surgicel has been placed behind – on the concave side of the anterior loop of the ICA into the sella in front of the PCP – and venous bleeding has been stopped.

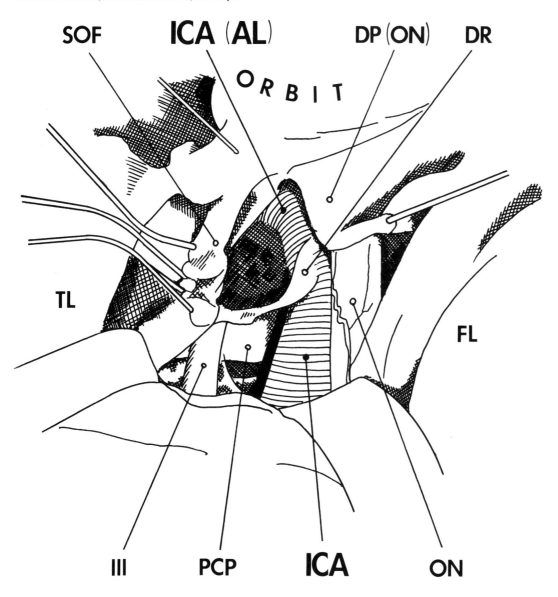

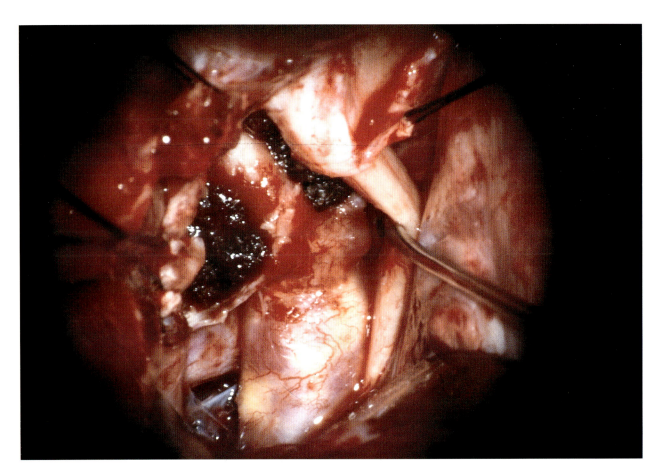

Fig. 118. The distal dural ring around the ICA proximal to the ophthalmic artery has been cut and the opthalmic artery can be visualized through retraction of the ON. Further dissection of the anterior loop of the ICA in the anteromedial triangle has been performed. Surgicel has been put on both sides of the ICA. Venous bleeding has been stopped

SOF   ICA (AL)   DP (ON)   OA

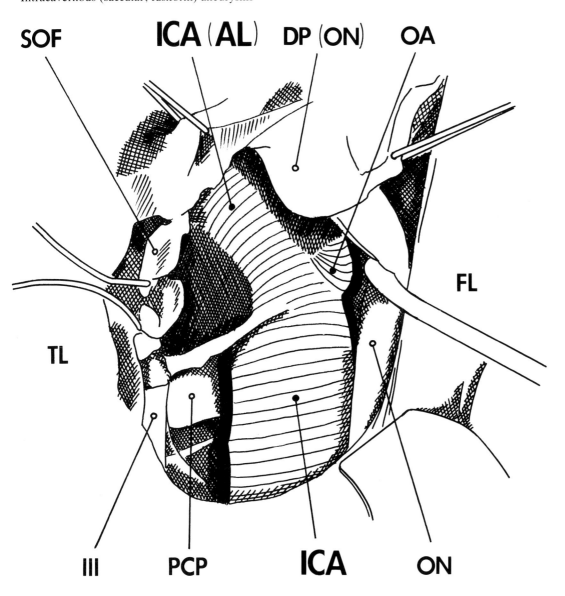

TL

FL

III   PCP   ICA   ON

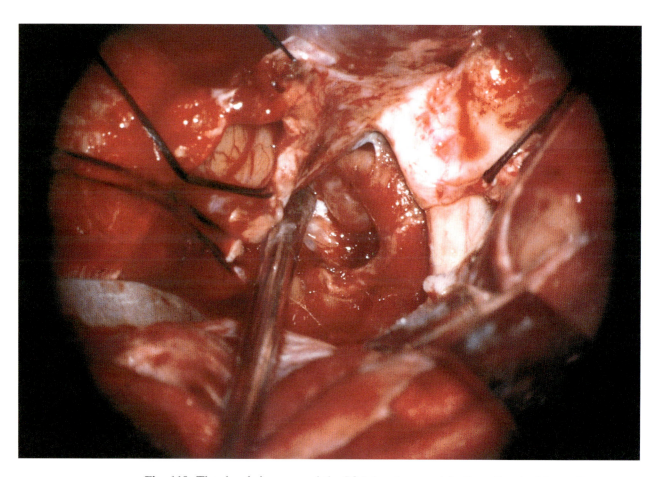

Fig. 119. The dural ring around the ICA has been cut further. Surgicel from the concave side of the anterior loop of the ICA has been removed and the aneurysm projecting backwards can be visualized. The whole extent of the anterior loop of the ICA and a part of the horizontal segment of the ICA in the CS is shown. Note: A part of the proximal ring around the carotid artery is still in place

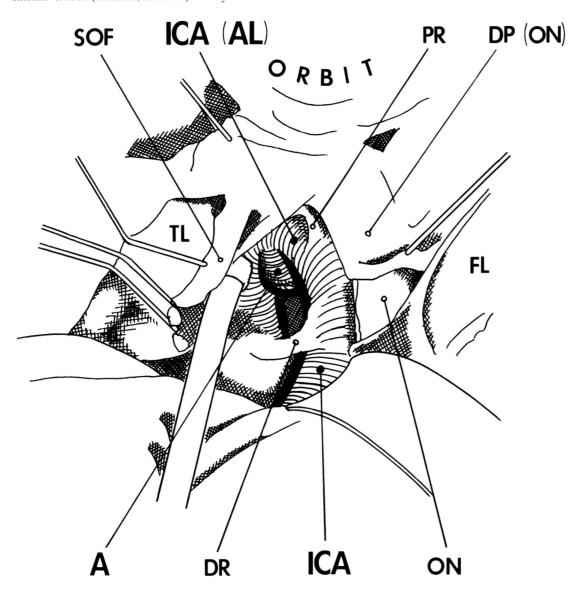

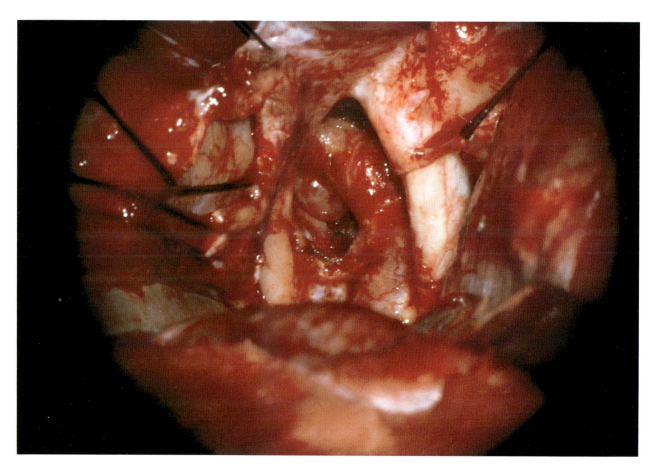

Fig. 120. The proximal ring around the ICA in the anteromedial triangle has been cut circumferentially around. The anterior loop of the ICA in the anteromedial triangle can be visualized completely. The aneurysm on the posterior aspect of the anterior loop of the ICA has been isolated and is shown in its entirety. A part of the horizontal segment of the ICA in the CS under the IIIrd nerve, which has been dissected further toward the SOF, can be seen. Some of the dural ring around the ICA in the lateral aspect is still in place

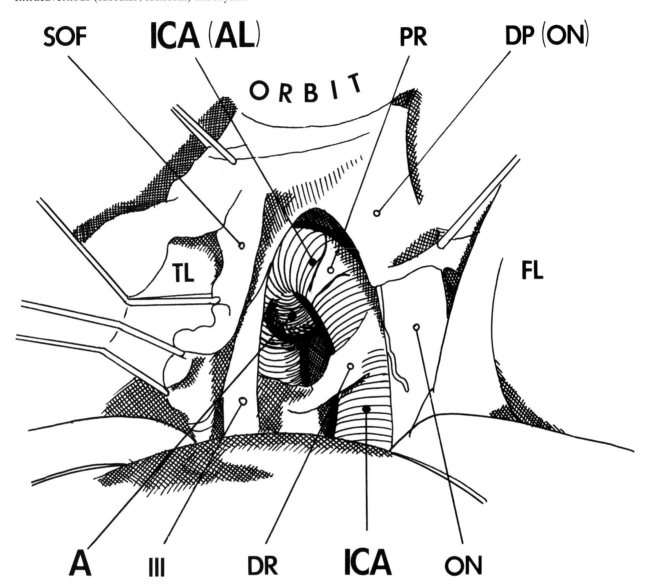

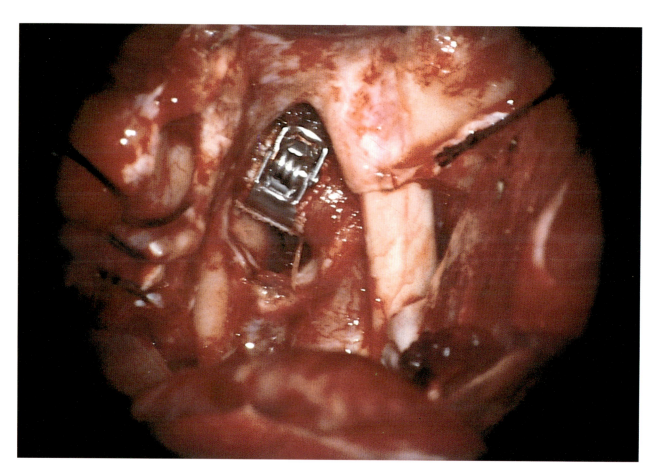

Fig. 121. A ring clip has been placed around the aneurysm and the ICA and in this way the aneurysm has been fixed. The whole anterior loop of the ICA, a part of the horizontal segment of the ICA in the CS, as well as the ICA intradurally, can be seen. The clip touches neither the ON nor the IIIrd nerve

SOF   ICA (AL)   DP (ON)   ON

ORBIT

TL

FL

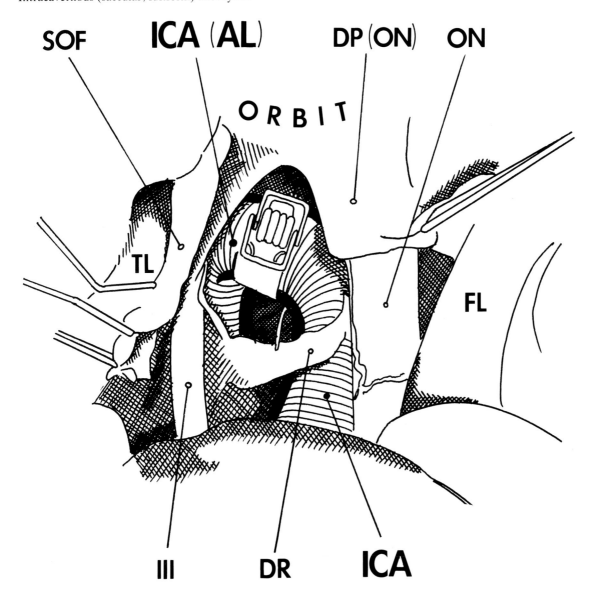

III   DR   ICA

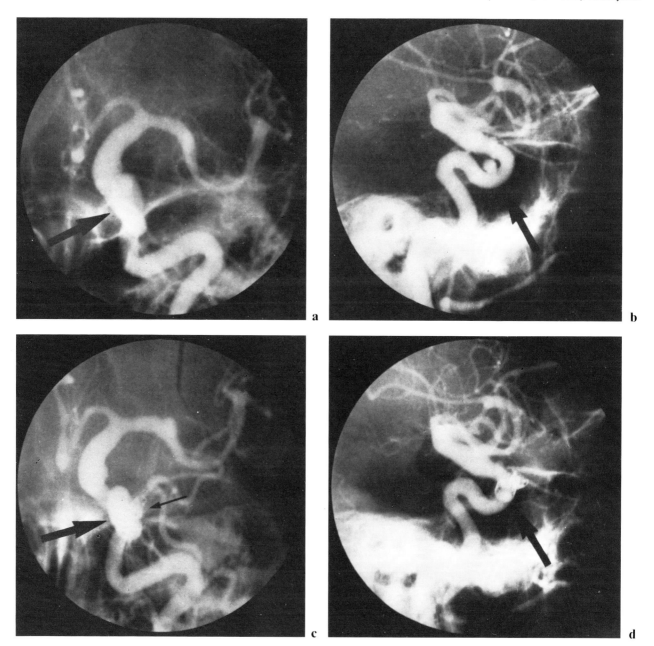

Fig. 122. Left carotid angiograms of the same patient as presented in Figs. 115–121, anteroposterior views (**a, c**) and lateral views (**b, d**). **a, b** Preoperative angiograms showing a small intracavernous ICA aneurysm on the posterior aspect of the anterior loop of the ICA. **c, d** Postoperative angiograms showing a ring clip around the anterior loop of the ICA in the CS, and no aneurysm

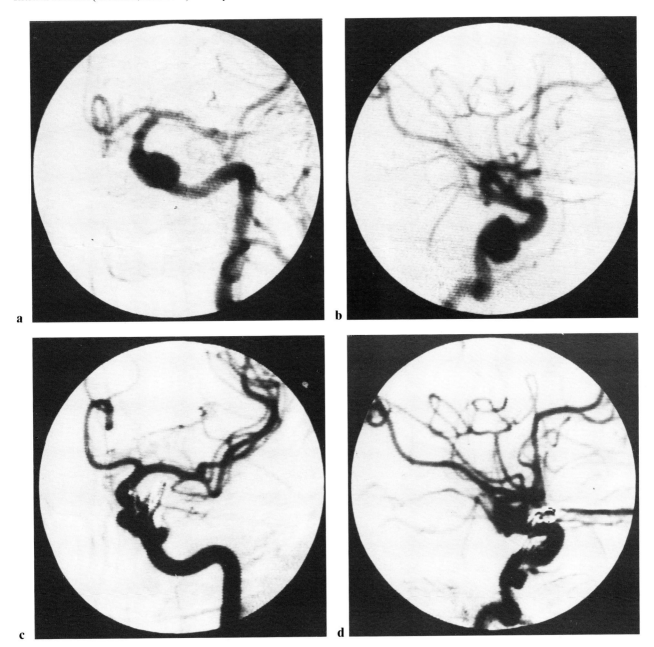

Fig. 123. Left carotid angiograms, anteroposterior views (**a, c**) and lateral views (**b, d**). **a, b** Preoperative angiograms showing a large intracavernous aneurysm on the medial loop and horizontal portion of the ICA in the CS. **c, d** Postoperative angiograms showing a clip and a small remnant of the aneurysm close to the lateral ring of the ICA in the CS. The remnant of the aneurysm has not increased in size over the last three years and the patient is symptom-free

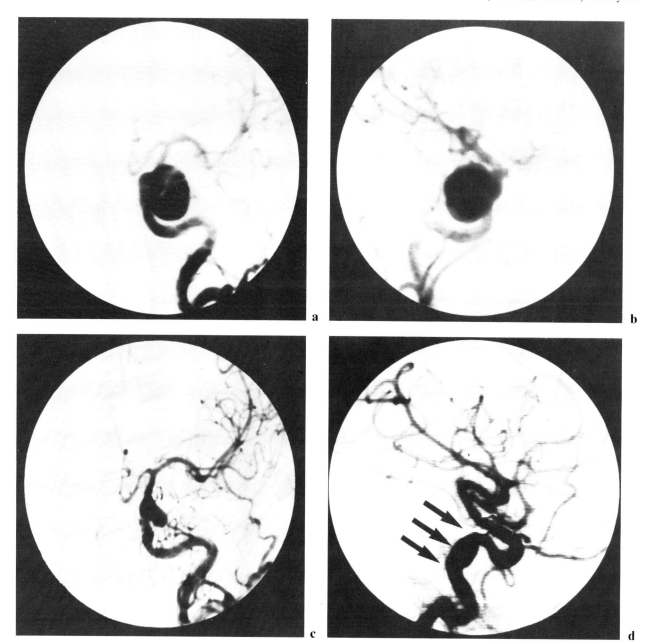

Fig. 124. Left carotid angiograms, anteroposterior views (**a, c**) and lateral views (**b, d**). **a, b** Preoperative angiograms showing a large intracavernous aneurysm causing severe headache and pain in the area of V1 and V2, as well as diplopia due to partial paresis of the VIth nerve. **c, d** Postoperative angiograms showing a slightly wider ICA at the site where the aneurysm was resected. The ICA was reconstructed by interrupted sutures and reinforced at the peripheral end of the neck of the aneurysm by a small Yasargil clip. Symptoms and signs disappeared completely within three months after surgery

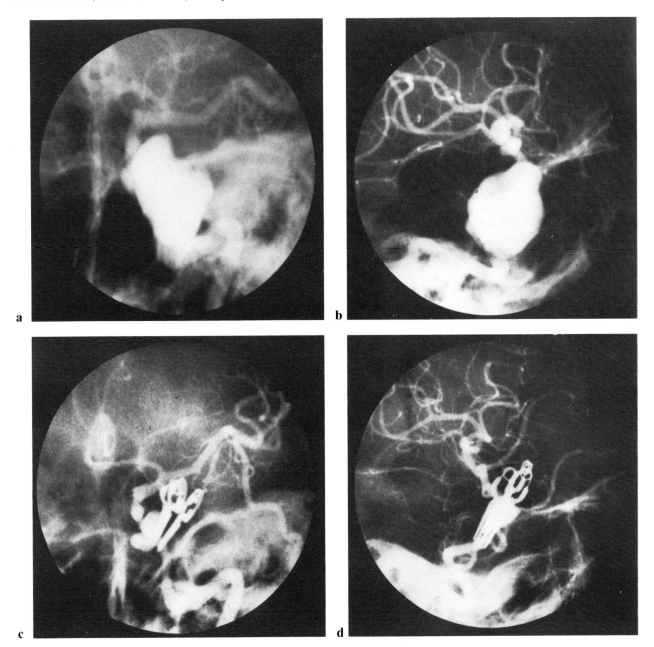

Fig. 125. Left carotid angiograms, anteroposterior views (**a, c**) and lateral views (**b, d**). **a, b** Preoperative angiograms showing a giant, partially thrombosed intracavernous aneurysm of the ICA which originated from the whole anterior loop of the ICA in the CS. **c, d** Postoperative angiograms showing three clips on the aneurysm. The aneurysm was entered and the blood clot removed. The neck of the aneurysm was cut and occluded by two Yasargil clips. The ICA together with the blades of these two clips was wrapped circumferentially around with musline tissue and the edges of the musline were fixed with a third clip. The third clip protects the first two clips from slipping from the neck of the aneurysm. The patient, who suffered from severe pain in the area of V1 and V2, and who had paresis of the IIIrd, IVth, and VIth nerve, was symptom-free six months after surgery and there has been no recurrence of symptoms

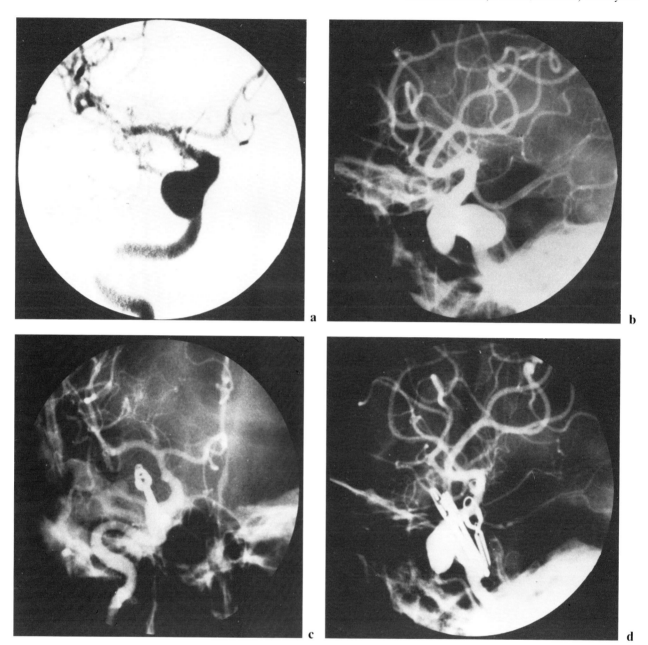

Fig. 126. Right carotid angiograms, anteroposterior views (**a, c**) and lateral views (**b, d**). **a, b** Preoperative angiograms showing an aneurysm on the horizontal segment and on the medial loop of the ICA in the CS. **c, d** Postoperative angiograms showing three clips on the intracavernous ICA aneurysm in the CS. The shadow peripheral to the clips represents an unusually long, irregular anterior loop of the ICA

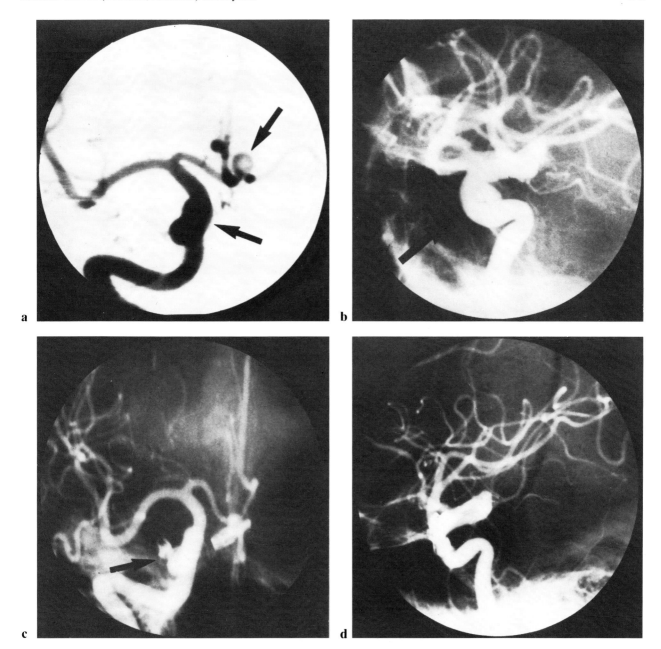

Fig. 127. Right carotid angiograms, anteroposterior views (**a, c**) and lateral views (**b, d**). **a, b** Preoperative angiograms showing an aneurysm of the ACoA and a small aneurysm on the posterior side of the anterior loop of the intracavernous ICA in the CS. **c, d** Postoperative angiograms showing a clip on the ACoA aneurysm and a ring clip around the aneurysm and the anterior loop of the intracavernous ICA in the CS. The patient was admitted to hospital because of a SAH caused by rupture of the aneurysm of the ACoA. Both aneurysms were clipped in one operation. From two weeks after surgery the patient has been symptom-free

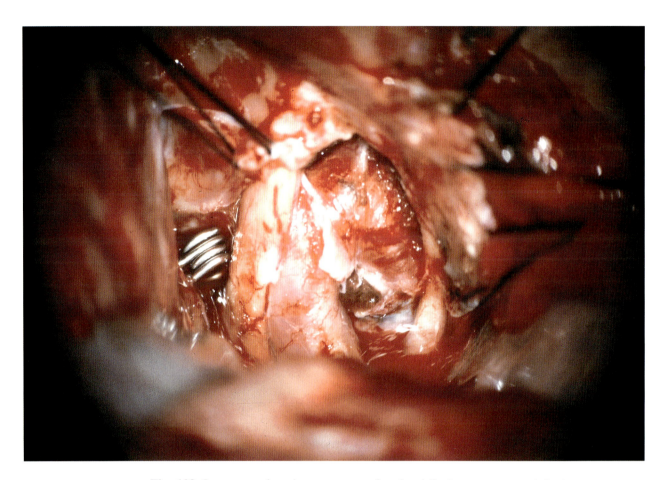

Fig. 128. Intraoperative view at surgery for the ACoA aneurysm and the intracavernous ICA aneurysm on the right side of the same patient as presented in Fig. 127. The ACoA aneurysm has been clipped, and a part of the clip can be seen on the medial aspect of the right ON. On the lateral aspect of the ON in the anteromedial triangle, the anterior loop of the ICA in the CS is shown. On the dorsal aspect of the anterior loop of the ICA a small aneurysm has been isolated. Lateral to the aneurysm, the IIIrd nerve can be seen

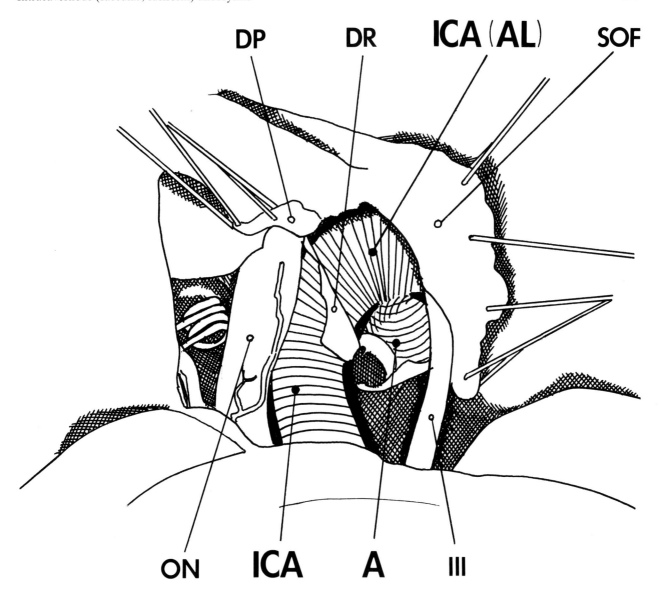

DP   DR   **ICA (AL)**   SOF

ON   **ICA**   A   III

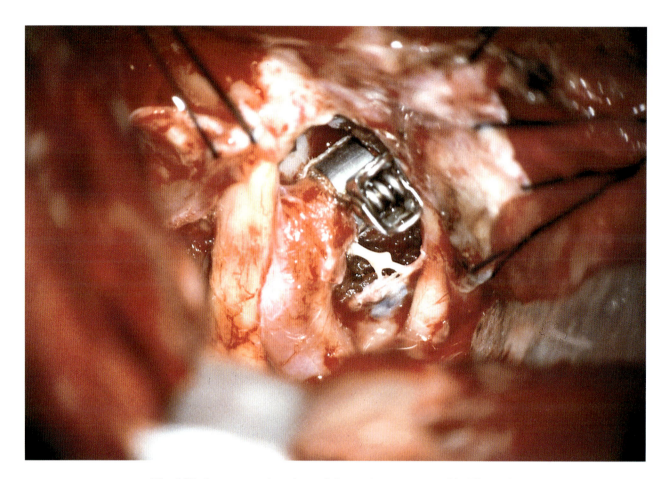

Fig. 129. Intraoperative view of the patient presented in Figs. 127 and 128. The anterior loop of the ICA in the CS is fully exposed. The ring clip has been placed around the anterior loop and the aneurysm. In this way, the aneurysm has been excluded. The ON is medial to the anterior loop of the ICA and the IIIrd nerve is lateral, and they are not in contact with the clip

ON   SOF

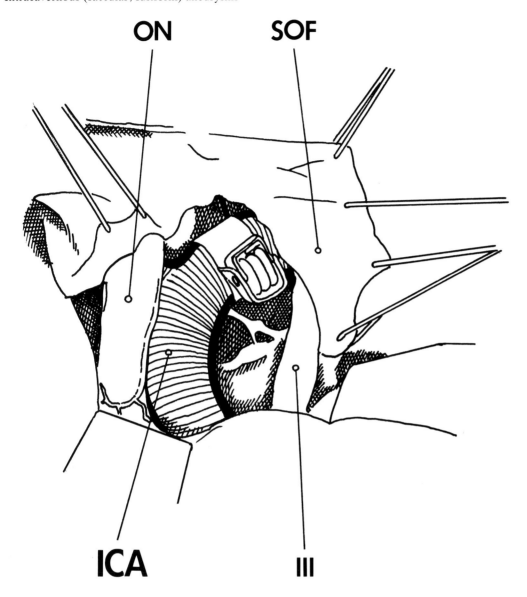

ICA   III

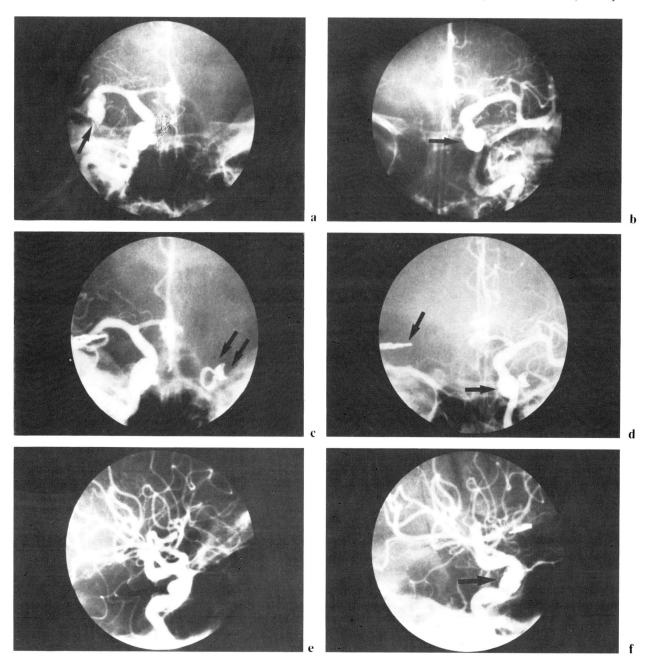

Fig. 130. Bilateral carotid angiograms, anteroposterior views (**a, d**) and lateral views (**e, f**). **a** Preoperative right carotid angiogram showing a MCA aneurysm, **b** left carotid angiogram showing a small intracavernous aneurysm. Postoperative angiograms show clips on the MCA (**c**) and on the ICA in the left CS (**d**). **e** Preoperative left carotid angiogram, lateral view, showing a small intracavernous aneurysm of the ICA on the dorsal aspect of the anterior loop, **f** postoperative angiogram showing a ring clip around the anterior loop of the ICA in the left CS. The patient was admitted to hospital after a SAH resulting from rupture of the right MCA aneurysm. The initial operation for the MCA aneurysm was performed in the acute stage one day post hemorrhage. Two weeks later, when the patient was symptom-free, the second operation was performed for the intracavernous ICA aneurysm in the left CS. From one month after the second operation, the patient has been symptom-free

4.2 Traumatic intracavernous aneurysms

In general, traumatic intracavernous aneurysms are regarded as rare complications of craniocerebral trauma with a skull base fracture. The relationship of the ICA to the skull base bony structures as well as the architecture of the bony structures adjacent to the ICA explain why most of the traumatic intracavernous ICA aneurysms occur at the anterior loop of the ICA. The lateral bony wall of the sphenoid sinus, which is on the medial aspect of the anterior loop of the ICA, is very thin and can easily be fractured (Figs. 52–55). On the other hand, the ACP, which is on the lateral aspect of the anterior loop of the ICA, is much bulkier and cannot be easily fractured (Figs. 42 and 43). In addition, the anterior loop of the ICA is fixed to the surrounding bony structures by two rings – the dural ring and the proximal ring – and with a thin, fibrous layer covering most of the lateral and anterior aspects of the anterior loop of the ICA between these two rings (Figs. 44 and 48–52). Since the bone on the medial aspect of the anterior loop of the ICA is thinner and easily fractured, it is clear that lesions of the artery wall will most likely occur on the medial aspect of the anterior loop of the ICA. This is the reason why most traumatic intracavernous aneurysms of the ICA are located on the anterior loop of the ICA and why most of them project downwards and anteriorly. Another traumatic lesion of the lateral wall of the sphenoid sinus adjacent to the medial aspect of the anterior loop of the ICA may result from a transsphenoidal approach to the pituitary tumor (Figs. 52–54).

Traumatic intracavernous ICA aneurysms can also be located on any other segment of the ICA at the skull base. However, when a traumatic intracavernous aneurysm is not located at the anterior loop of the ICA, it is usually not a consequence of a skull base fracture, but of a direct stab wound, in most cases through the orbit and the SOF. In such cases, it is more likely that the horizontal segment of the ICA from the lateral to the medial loop will be injured. Stab wounds to the ICA in the CS will most probably result in a CCF rather than in a traumatic intracavernous aneurysm. It should be pointed out that traumatic intracavernous aneurysms are actually false aneurysms. This means that the so-called aneurysm wall is not a thin outpouching of the arterial wall, but of tissue surrounding the artery. This also explains why injury to the ICA wall, either by a bony spicula or any sharp object causing a stab wound sometimes results in a false aneurysm, and, at other times, in a CCF. It is only the fibrous structure surrounding the artery which ruptures allowing arterial blood from the injured ICA to enter the venous channels of the CS. In severe trauma, it is more likely that injury to the artery wall will be more extensive in both directions: on both the longitudinal axis of the artery and the circumference of the artery wall. In the most severe cases, the ICA can be completely torn. It is then also very likely that the CS facing the intradural compartments will be injured and that there could be a coexistent SAH. In the great majority of cases with mild trauma, the traumatic intracavernous aneurysm is located close to the fracture, that is, on the anteromedial aspect of the wall of the anterior loop of the ICA. Only exceptionally are traumatic aneurysms located on the posterior or lateral aspect of the anterior loop of the ICA. However, it is possible that, in a patient with a pre-existent small saccular intracavernous aneurysm on the posterior or lateral aspect of the anterior loop of the ICA, following trauma this pre-existent aneurysm can be transformed into a larger traumatic aneurysm, or, if the wall of the ICA is injured on the anterior loop on the anteromedial side, a further traumatic aneurysm can occur.

In most cases of traumatic ICA intracavernous aneurysms there is also loss of vision on the side of the aneurysm. Blindness in the ipsilateral eye is ascribed to a lesion of the ON in the optic canal due to a skull base fracture. The latter causes injury to the artery wall which results in a traumatic aneurysm. Severe arterial nose bleeding, ipsilateral loss of vision, and a skull base fracture at the site of a traumatic aneurysm compose the classical triad originally described by Maurer [27] and subsequently by other authors [1, 2]. These symptoms call for urgent treatment.

The ideal treatment of traumatic intracavernous aneurysms is: (a) reconstruction of the arterial wall by clipping and wrapping the artery and the clip(s) with musline tissue, and by placing an additional clip over the musline, (b) by placing a ring clip over the aneurysm and the artery, or by suturing the artery wall with interrupted sutures, (c) by grafting. Or, if none of the above methods is possible, by extra-intra-anastomosis and occlusion of the ICA proximal and distal to the traumatic aneurysm.

For direct reconstruction of the ICA wall in traumatic aneurysms, the described general approach to the CS is mandatory. The ICA should be exposed in the petrous bone through the posterolateral triangle to obtain necessary proximal control and to enable insertion of the graft. Only when the posterior loop of the ICA is properly exposed, is the dura incised and dissection of the ICA in the anteromedial triangle is commenced. The method of repair is chosen according to the location and extent of the lesion of the artery wall.

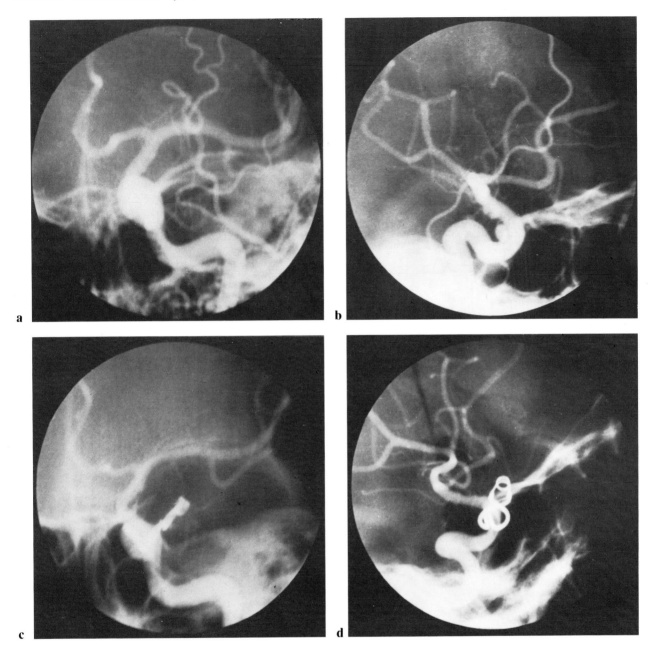

Fig. 131. Left carotid angiograms, anteroposterior views (**a, c**) and lateral views (**b, d**). **a, b** Preoperative angiograms showing a small traumatic aneurysm on the posteromedial side on the anterior loop of the ICA in the CS. **c, d** Postoperative angiograms showing a fenestrated clip on the aneurysm on the anterior loop of the ICA in the CS. Note that the blades of the clip hold both part of the arterial wall and surrounding tissue so that the false aneurysm is completely exluded and patency of the ICA is sufficiently preserved

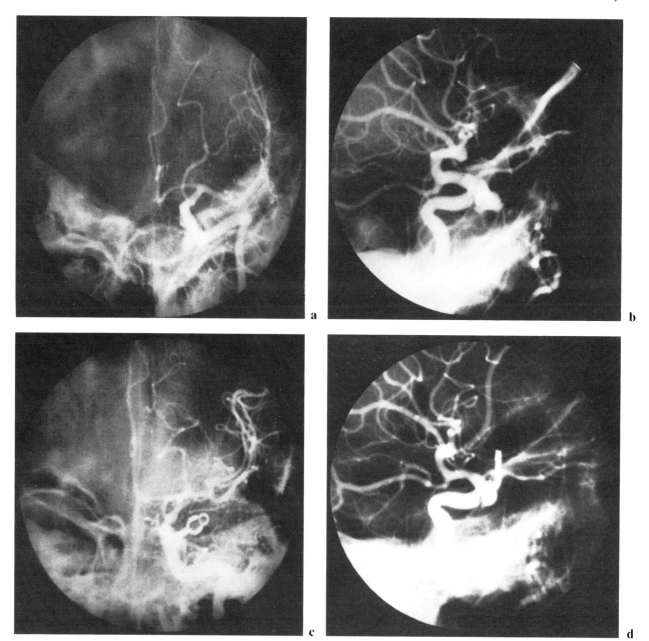

Fig. 132. Left carotid angiograms, anteroposterior views (**a, c**) and lateral views (**b, d**). **a, b** Preoperative angiograms showing a small traumatic aneurysm projecting anteromedially downwards into the sphenoid sinus. Note the rough, irregular surface of the aneurysm which shows the blood clot around the aneurysm in the sphenoid sinus. **c, d** Postoperative angiograms showing a clip on the neck of the aneurysm on the anterior aspect of the anterior loop of the ICA in the CS. A false aneurysm is still present beside the clip. The anterior loop was wrapped circumferentially around with musline. The clip was put on the musline, so that the free ends of the musline are tightly secured with the clip. The pseudoaneurysm, which is still present is inside the cuff. In this way, further bleeding is impossible. The patient, who had four severe arterial nose bleeds preoperatively, has been symptom-free ever since the surgery

4.3 Carotid-cavernous fistulas

It is generally agreed that carotid-cavernous fistulas (CCFs) are abnormal communications between the ICA and the CS. The same is true for abnormal communications between the branches of the ICA and/or branches of the external carotid artery (ECA) and the CS. CCFs are either a result of trauma, or they may arise spontaneously. Most traumatic CCFs are a result of skull base fractures, however, they may also be caused by penetrating injuries such as knife or gun shot wounds (Fig. 133). The injury to the ICA and abnormal communication between the ICA and CS in traumatic CCFs is in most cases located on the segment of the ICA between the lateral and proximal rings of the ICA (Figs. 47–51). The location of the injury to the ICA on its longitudinal axis or its circumference depends on the location of the skull base fracture or the trajectory of the wounding object. In rare cases, however, when the lesion of the ICA is caused by avulsion of the MHT or the ILT, the bone fracture might be relatively distant to the site of injury of the ICA.

A relatively large number of CCFs occur spontaneously but the majority are caused by rupture of an intracavernous ICA aneurysm into the venous compartments of the CS [5, 31. 32, 39, 46, 53]. The etiology of most spontaneous CCFs is speculative [26, 30, 46]. Rupture of the small branches of the ICA and ECA into the CS in spontaneous CCFs can be caused by various factors, such as arterial hypertension, atherosclerotic vascular disease, hypertension associated with pregnancy, minor trauma, straining, or collagen vascular disease [11, 30, 34, 40, 45, 46, 49, 54].

On anatomical and radiographic grounds, four types of CCFs have been proposed, as follows:
a) direct shunts between the ICA and the CS
b) dural shunts between the meningeal branches of the ICA and the CS
c) dural shunts between the meningeal branches of the ECA and the CS, and
d) dural shunts between the meningeal branches of both the ICA and the ECA and the CS [38].

It is important to know, whether a CCF is a high-flow or a low-flow fistula. The majority of high-flow CCFs, most of which are traumatic in origin, require more prompt treatment than low-flow CCFs. The characteristic clinical picture of a high-flow CCF is represented by the triad of pulsating exophthalmos with ocular chemosis, a subjective and very disturbing, audible bruit synchronous with the heart beat, and visual impairment or loss on the side of the CCF. In cases of spontaneous CCFs, the clinical picture is very mild initially but may become severe as the fistula increases in size. In such cases visual deterioration, obtrusive diplopia, an intolerable bruit and/or headache and proptosis with corneal exposure call for urgent treatment as for high-flow CCFs.

There is no vascular pathology of the central nervous system in which so much controversy has remained until recently with regard to the best method of treatment. The detachable balloon catheter technique plays a very important, if not the most important, role in the treatment of high-flow CCFs [6, 43, 53]. The direct surgical approach to the CS in the treatment of CCFs was first performed in 1936 by Browder [4] and subsequently refined by Parkinson [36]. In subsequent years, other surgical methods were introduced, among which inserting various thrombogenic materials into the CCF was the most popular [29]. Finally, a safe and rather easy direct microsurgical approach to the CS was introduced [7].

Whatever the method of treatment of CCFs, it should provide for the exclusion of the fistula and maintenance of the patency of the ICA. If this is achieved, the troublesome bruit will disappear and reduction of the exophthalmos will follow, oculomotor function will improve, and in cases where the visual function of the eye is still present, the diplopia will disappear.

Recently, it has been agreed that the detachable balloon catheter technique and the direct surgical approach to the CS are no longer competing, but complementary modalities in the treatment of CCFs.

For the direct approach to CCFs the surgical technique for the epidural stage and dural incision is as described in Chap. 2.

Sufficient exposure of the ICA in both the posterolateral and anteromedial triangles is essential as in surgery for intracavernous aneurysms. The next step is dissection of the IIIrd and the IVth nerve from the entry point to the lateral wall of the CS towards the SOF. Whenever possible, these two nerves should be dissected without entering the CS and with necessary occlusion of the intracavernous segment of the ICA. Following complete dissection of the IIIrd and the IVth nerves, temporary clips are placed on the posterior and anterior loops of the ICA and the ICA is dissected from the anterior loop along the horizontal segment toward the medial loop and finally (when necessary) from the medial toward the lateral loop. In high-flow traumatic CCFs it is usually necessary to reconstruct the ICA wall with interrupted sutures (Fig. 136). In some of these CCFs it is possible to exclude the fistula and reconstruct the ICA with a ring clip (Figs. 135 and 137). The reconstruction of the ICA with interrupted sutures and/or clipping is also necessary in most CCFs resulting from rupture of a preexisting intracavernous aneurysm. In the great majority of low-flow spontaneous CCFs it is possible to exclude the fistula using bipolar coagulation and by packing the CS around the ICA with Surgicel or pieces of muscle and fibrin glue. In some cases of high-flow CCFs, either traumatic or spontaneous, following intracavernous aneurysm rupture, when the defect of the ICA wall cannot be repaired by direct suturing or by applying ring or straight clips, reconstruction of the ICA by the insertion of a vein graft from the posterior to the anterior loop is necessary. Such a situation should be anticipated (Fig. 133) and a vein graft should be prepared at the beginning of the operation. Precise angiographic location of the CCF is mandatory in each case when surgery is planned (Fig. 134). Precise localization of a CCF with angiographic studies is of great help in the dissection of the intracavernous ICA and it significantly shortens the time of occlusion of the ICA. Preoperative cross studies from the left to the right carotid system, and retrograde studies from the vertebral to the carotid system towards the intracavernous lesion, are of paramount importance and dictate the maximum possible period of temporary occlusion of the ICA or, on the other hand, may indicate that permanent occlusion of the ICA is possible, if for some reason reconstruction cannot be carried out.

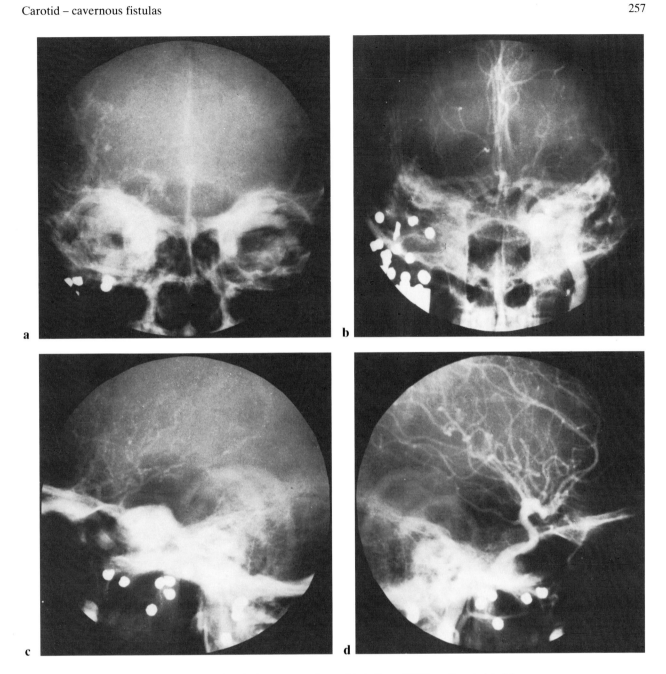

Fig. 133. Right carotid angiograms (**a, c**) demonstrating a high-flow CCF on the right side extending to the left side, barely visible right intracranial arterial tree, and several small-shots in the extracranial and skull base areas on the right side. Left carotid angiograms (**b, d**) demonstrating normal ICA in the CS, normal arterial tree on the left side with good cross flow to the right side and small-shots.

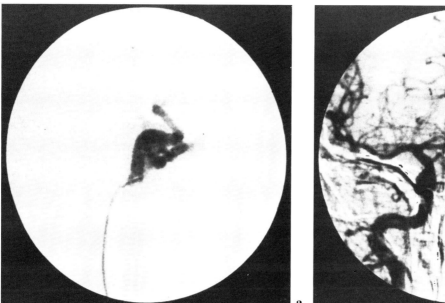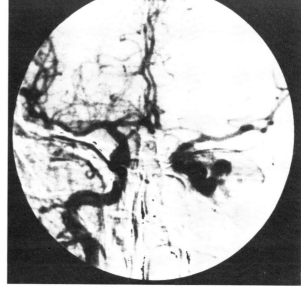

Fig. 134. a The catheter is shown in the left intracavernous segment of the ICA and the CCF, located on the horizontal segment of the ICA in the lateral view. **b** Right carotid angiogram with good cross filling of the left carotid arterial tree and retrograde filling of the CCF in AP view is shown

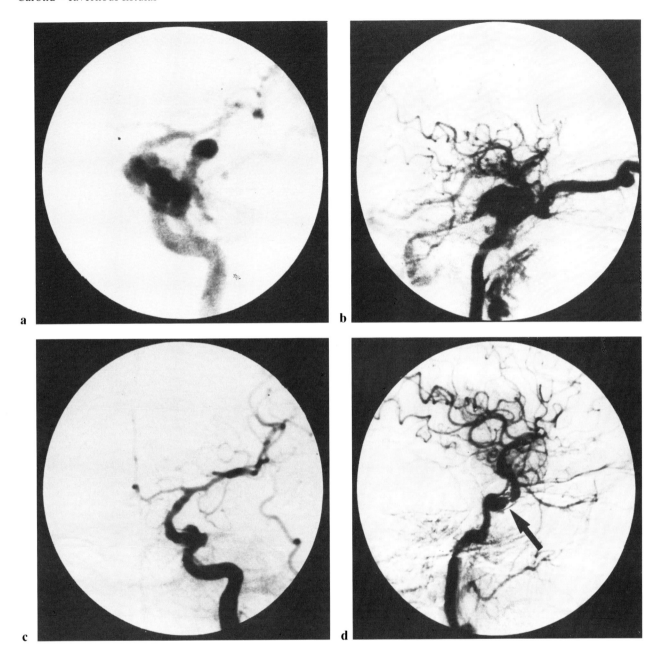

Fig. 135. Left carotid angiograms, anteroposterior views (**a, c**) and lateral views (**b, d**). **a, b:** Preoperative angiograms showing a large CCF with the major draining vein to the orbit and through the SPS as well as through the skull base (**b**). **c, d:** Postoperative angiograms showing normal intracavernous segment of the ICA and a ring clip on the horizontal segment of the intracavernous ICA (**d**)

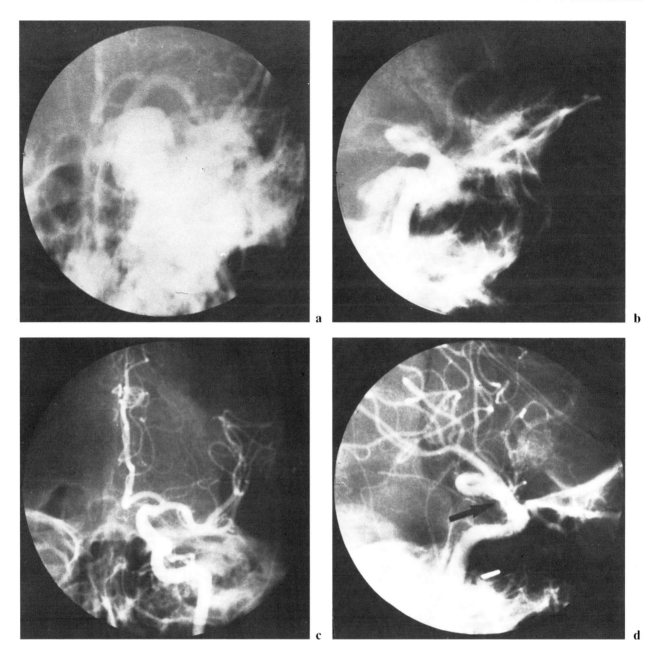

Fig. 136. Left carotid angiograms, anteroposterior views (**a, c**) and lateral views (**b, d**). **a, b** Preoperative angiograms showing a large CCF on the horizontal segment and anterior loop of the intracavernous ICA. **c,d** Postoperative angiograms showing a normal intracavernous ICA and no CCF. The defect of the ICA has been repaired with interrupted sutures

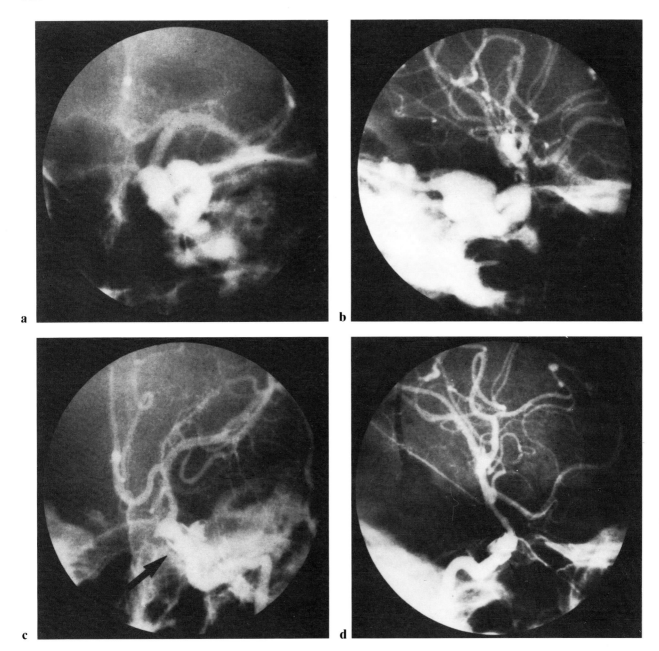

Fig. 137. Left carotid angiograms, anteroposterior views (**a, c**) and lateral views (**b, d**). **a, b** Preoperative angiograms showing a large CCF on the anterior loop of the intracavernous ICA. The main drainage is in a posterior direction. **c, d** Postoperative angiograms showing a ring clip at the anterior loop of the intracavernous ICA, and no CCF. Vasospasm is seen along the whole intradural segment of the ICA

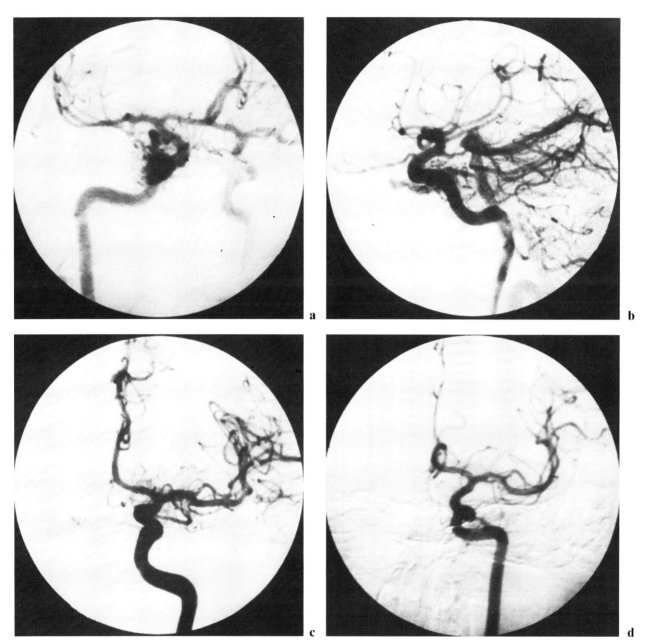

Fig. 138. a Right carotid angiogram in the AP view shows a CCF on the right side and good cross flow to the left carotid system. **b** Vertebral angiogram in the lateral view shows good filling of the right carotid system and CCF on the right side. **c** Left carotid angiogram in the AP view shows an intracavernous branch originating from the MHT of the left ICA and feeding the CCF on the right side. **d** Left carotid angiogram postoperatively in the AP view is normal

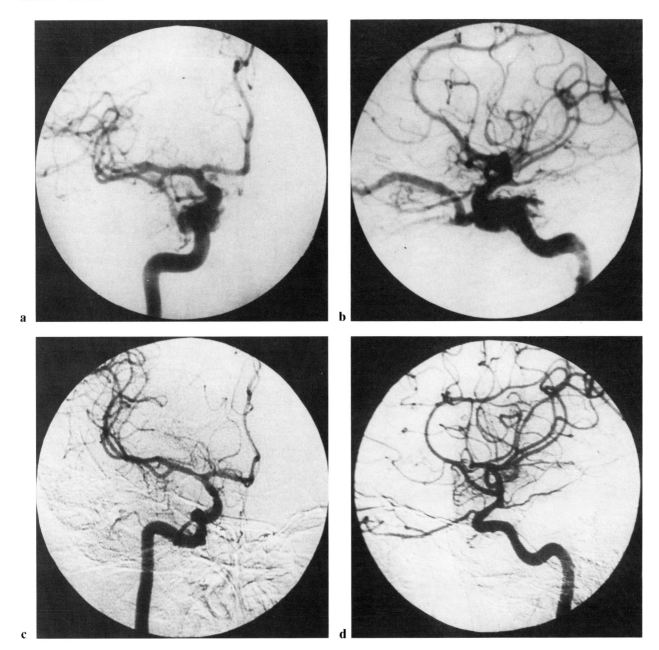

Fig. 139. Right carotid angiograms, anteroposterior views (**a, c**) and lateral views (**b, d**) of the same patient as presented in Fig. 138. **a, b** Preoperative angiograms showing a CCF located on the horizontal segment of the intracavernous ICA with engorgement of the ophthalmic vein. **b, d** Postoperative angiograms showing no fistula. Feeders from the left and right ICA to the fistula were excluded by bipolar coagulation and the right CS was packed with Surgicel and pieces of muscle

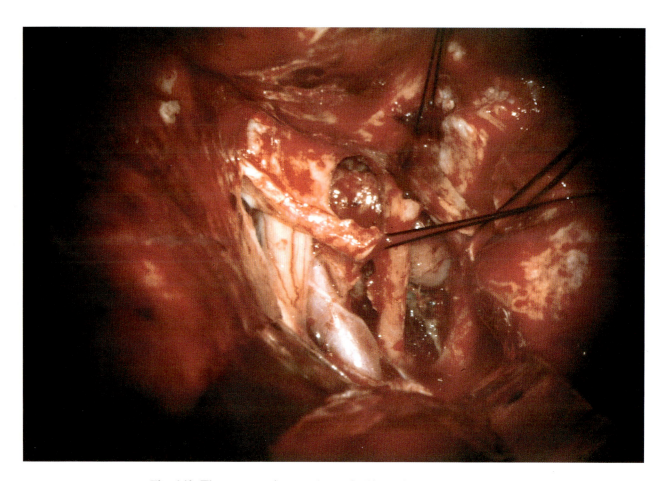

Fig. 140. The same patient as shown in Figs. 138 and 139. The right CS has been explored. The ICA has been dissected along the entire anterior loop, horizontal segment and medial loop. The CCF has been excluded by bipolar coagulation of feeders from the right and left ICA to the CCF

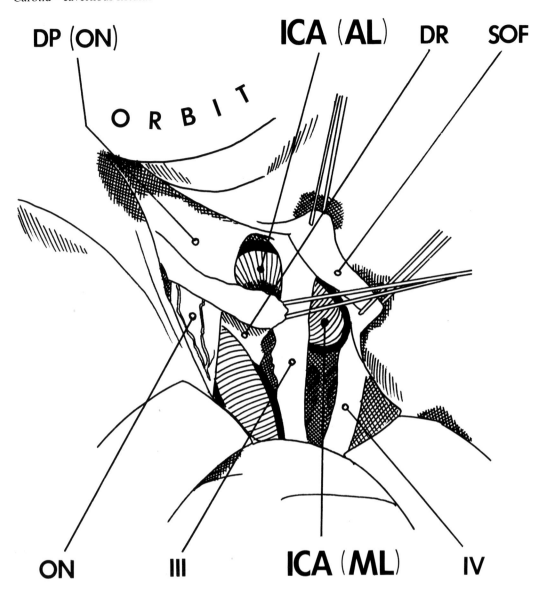

DP (ON) ORBIT ICA (AL) DR SOF

ON III ICA (ML) IV

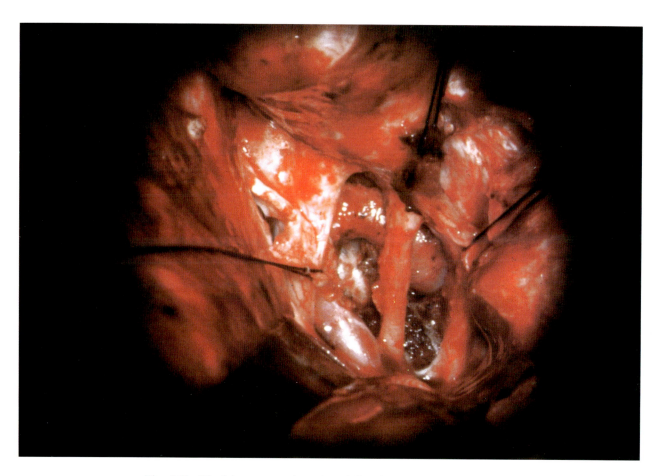

Fig. 141. Final intraoperative view following the complete exclusion of the CCF in the patient presented in Figs. 138–140. Note Surgicel on the medial aspect of the medial loop of the ICA. The bottom of the sella is clearly shown. The medial loop, the horizontal segment and the anterior loop of the intracavernous ICA are presented in the right CS. The IIIrd and the IVth nerve have been dissected. The approach into the entire CS was possible through the anteromedial and paramedial triangles

DP (ON)   ICA (AL)   SOF

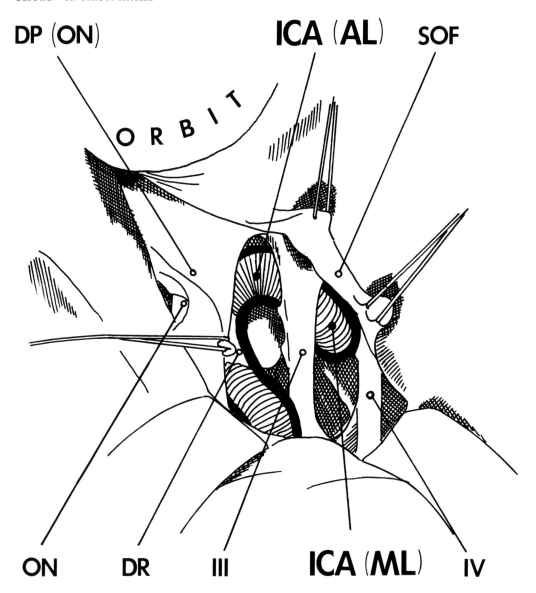

ON   DR   III   ICA (ML)   IV

5 Cavernous sinus tumors

Tumors in the CS may occur in children, are most frequent in the middle-aged, but still occur quite frequently in the older-age group. Female patients outnumber male patients by 2:1. Over 90% of tumors occurring in, or invading the CS are benign meningiomas. Intracavernous tumors in children are, in most cases, neurinomas of nerve V. Many other benign tumors may affect the CS, among which the most frequent are rather invasive but benign tumors of the pituitary gland. Malignant tumors of the CS include sarcomas and carcinomas from the surrounding areas, as well as other malignant tumors. Even metastases can be found in the CS.

Symptoms and signs in patients with CS tumors are: headache, paresis of nerves III through VI, exophthalmos, ophthalmoplegia, neuralgic pain in V1 and/or V2. Headache is usually mild at the onset of the disease and in most cases remains unchanged throughout the course although subsequently additional symptoms and signs develop. In a relatively large number of patients, headache is accompanied quite early by diplopia due to paresis of nerves III, IV, and/or VI. Exophthalmos is rare, and ophthalmoplegia is only occasionally seen prior to admittance of the patient to hospital. Severe neuralgic pain in V1 and/or V2 areas on the side of the CS tumor indicates the location of a benign tumor in the SOF or a malignant tumor elsewhere in the CS and irritation of the branches of the Vth nerve or the GG itself. Various pathological processes in the CS can cause the same symptoms and signs [13, 50, 52] and so typical clinical patterns for each of the CS lesions have been described in detail [15, 16, 19, 20, 22, 24, 28, 48]. Since CT and MRI have become available, the diagnosis of CS lesions has become much easier. At present, clinical pictures for different CS lesions do not necessarily tell exactly what the lesion is but justify the need for CT and/or MRI scanning. CT or MRI examinations without contrast media can easily give a false negative result if the lesion is small and isodense with blood. It is also wrong to try to predict the histological nature of the lesion only on the basis of CT scan or MRI. When the diagnosis of an infection in the orbit and the CS is highly probable, a transorbital needle biopsy can be useful [44].

Four vessel angiography and cross studies definitely differentiate tumors from vascular lesions and provide important data on changes of the ICA in the CS on the side of the tumor as well as changes of the other intracranial arteries. Whenever the ICA in the CS is displaced and/or stenotic, cross studies and ICA occlusion test with the balloon catheter are mandatory preoperatively. The exact data on changes of the ICA encroached by the tumor in the CS define the strategy of resection of the tumor from the ICA. While narrowing of the ICA in the CS usually does not imply stenosis, but invasion of the tumor into the artery wall, it is advisable to leave the tumor around the artery in areas where angiographic changes are shown, in all cases in which cross flows are not good and/or ICA occlusion test is positive. In such cases, additional gamma knife radiosurgery is preferable shortly after direct microsurgical subtotal resection of the tumor.

EMG studies of periocular muscles and of muscles innervated by the Vth nerve are necessary preoperatively. They provide a valuable estimation of the condition of these muscles. Peroperative monitoring is useful but is far from being a substitute for the surgeon's knowledge of the anatomy. In patients with a tumor located in the anterior portion of the CS, around the ACP, and in those with possible invasion of the tumor into the optic canal, conventional perimetry studies and visual evoked potentials should be recorded.

On the basis of the results obtained preoperatively, it is possible to predict more objectively the changes that might ensue from the manipulation of nerves III through VI and the ICA during the dissection. After the assessment of ACoA and PCoA patencies and after the ICA occlusion test, one can anticipate the patient's tolerance of possible temporary or permanent occlusion of the ICA on the side of the CS tumor in patients with obvious changes to the ICA, manifested as a narrowing of the diameter as a result of invasion of the tumor into the wall of the artery.

From a practical point of view, the origin of the tumor, as well as its location, play the main role in surgery and determine to a great extent when and if a lesion can be surgically completely excised without leaving permanent neurological deficits.

A tumor, usually a meningioma, originating elsewhere around the CS can easily invade the CS through the anatomical openings through which the nerves III through VI enter the wall of the CS. It is obvious that a meningioma located primarily at the tip of the PCP and in the area of the oculomotor trigone will easily enter the canal of the IIIrd nerve (Fig. 142) and then from the canal through the thin medial, inner wall of the canal into the CS. In this way, tumors arising at the ACP and PCP, on the lateral part of the diaphragm of the sella, at the anterior part of the edge of the tentorium, in the whole area of the oculomotor trigone, and in the areas of the tuberculum and dorsum sellae reach the CS through the oculomotor canal (Figs. 142–144). Meningiomas in these areas also usually invade the optic canal on one or both sides (Fig. 144). Bilateral invasion of the CS by these meningiomas occurs occasionally. A meningioma growing from the area of the oculomotor trigone along the oculomotor nerve through the canal into the CS also easily invades the lateral part of the sella in front of the PCP and accompanies the ON into the optic canal anteriorly, while posteriorly it expands behind the PCP into the area of the inferomedial triangle (Figs. 154–156).

Meningiomas originating from the tentorial edge at the base of the paramedian and/or Parkinson's triangle and invading the CS along the IVth and the Vth nerve also grow medialwards and caudalwards and reach the entry points of the IIIrd and the VIth nerves. Such meningiomas usually reach a large size in the CS, however, the more bulky part of the tumor remains in the posterior fossa and exerts severe compression on the brain stem (Figs. 158 and 162). These meningiomas should not be confused with petroclival meningiomas, for which the surgical approach is different and in which exploration of the CS is not needed.

Meningiomas invading the CS from the middle cranial fossa directly through the lateral wall of the CS are usually very large and may be located simultaneously in the middle, anterior and posterior cranial fossas (Fig. 179). These meningiomas grow right through the CS, and invade the sella and the optic canal. They have a very rich arterial blood supply and should be considered, because of their behaviour, as malignant tumors in spite of the histological characteristics which may not show any malignant features. After complete surgical excision of such a tumor additional irradiation is advisable (Fig. 178).

Invasive pituitary tumors may easily grow beyond the boundaries of the sella. When this is the case, such a tumor will either compress or invade the CS in a lateral direction. Whether the tumor from the sella compresses or invades the CS is determined by the membrane dividing the sella from parasellar compartments (Figs. 59–61). It is evident that a sellar tumor which has actually invaded the CS cannot be removed completely through a transsphenoidal approach. For this reason, it is better to choose "a priori" a transcranial approach and to remove the lesion totally from the CS and the sella in one session. The same procedure is advisable for craniopharyngiomas invading the CS from the sellar region.

The majority of tumors which originate in the CS itself are also meningiomas. Two rather important groups of tumors in the CS are neurinomas of the Vth nerve and chordomas. Whereas chordomas can easily be completely removed, this is not always the case with neurinomas of the Vth nerve, and is very difficult to achieve in cases of intracavernous meningiomas which occupy the whole CS and completely surround the ICA. In the latter situation, the artery wall is infiltrated by the tumor which blurs the cleavage line between the tumor and the surface of the artery. Consequently, it is impossible to safely completely remove the tumor without damaging the ICA wall. It is wiser to leave a layer of the tumor on the artery wall rather than to risk artery rupture during the postoperative period. However, in cases with a negative ICA occlusion test and good cross flow, resection of the ICA segment and complete removal of the tumor is prefered if the infiltration of the artery wall extends over a longer segment. In such cases, a vein graft is inserted between the posterior and distal loops of the ICA, and end-to-end and/or end-to-side anastomoses are performed with interrupted sutures. Grafting of the ICA should be performed to the extent that the whole length of the diseased ICA is excised. It is of paramount importance that the anastomosis of the proximal and distal stumps with a graft is performed in the healthy side of the ICA. If one is not in favor of grafting of the ICA in the case of surgical injury to the ICA while dissecting the tumor from its surface, it is better to occlude the artery proximally and distally than to risk a doubtful reconstruction of the surgical lesion in the diseased arterial wall since such a wall will not heal normally after the reconstruction, and rupture is very likely in the postoperative period.

The general surgical approach to all CS tumors is the same as described in Chap. 2.

In addition to that described, in the epidural phase of the operation for CS tumors, the second division of the trigeminal nerve has to be visualized in the bony canal beyond the CS, peripheral to the foramen rotundum in the canal of V2. The dissection of the ICA in the petrous bone in the posterolateral triangle is mandatory for all cases of intracavernous tumors even if the ICA in the CS does not show displacement or change in its shape. Proximal exposure of the ICA at the neck is not the same as exposure of the ICA in the petrous bone, which is necessary whenever grafting of the ICA might be contemplated. On the other hand, proximal catheter balloon occlusion of the ICA while performing end-to-end anastomosis between the posterior loop of the ICA and the proximal end of the venous graft is necessary for two reasons: injury to the ICA by the balloon is less probable than by temporary clips and, secondly, when the clips are not on the ICA close to the site of the anastomosis, there is more space available and the anastomosis can be more easily and better performed. Exploration of the ICA in the petrous bone can be omitted only in those cases in which one can be sure on the basis of CT and/or MRI, that the tumor involves only a minor portion of the CS and does not reach the intracavernous ICA. Only when the epidural phase of the operation is properly completed can the incision of the dura be started. The dural opening should be large enough to visualize the whole lateral wall of the CS, its transition to the orbital structures, the anteromedial triangle, the ON and posteriorly the dura overlying V3.

In cases in which the tumor enters the optic canal, the dura propria is incised along the longitudinal axis of the ON along its entire segment in the optic canal and, if necessary, through the annulus of Zinn (Figs. 148 and 150). Care must be taken not to damage the ophthalmic artery. In most cases of tumors in this area the dural ring around the carotid artery should be cut circumferentially around the ICA. The ICA can then be mobilized, the whole sellar space sufficiently visualized, and the tumor removed. The intercavernous sinuses can be easily visualized and occluded with Surgicel. If the tumor surrounds the anterior loop of the ICA it can be removed by this approach using only access through the anteromedial triangle. When the tumor extends beyond the anteromedial triangle and occupies the space around the horizontal segment of the ICA, dissection of the IIIrd nerve from its entry point into the lateral wall of the CS to the orbit should be performed. Dissection of the IIIrd nerve in its entire length is essential for access to the horizontal segment of the ICA through the paramedial triangle. Whenever access to intracavernous lesions is required through the paramedial triangle, the IVth nerve should also be dissected in its entire segment from the entry point into the lateral wall of the CS to the orbit in order to avoid its being damaged while dissecting the IIIrd nerve in its peripheral course, anterior to the anterior loop of the ICA and close to the orbit. With dissection of the ON, the IIIrd and the IVth nerve, and cutting of the dural ring around the ICA, the majority of tumors in this area can be completely removed (Figs. 143, 144 and 154). When a tumor is located more posteriorly and extends into the posterior fossa (Fig. 158), dissection of the IIIrd and IVth nerve is also required, and the tentorium is cut and the Vth nerve visualized in its course over the crest of the apex of the petrous bone towards Meckel's cave. The SPS is ligated or packed with Surgicel and the lateral wall of the CS is excised together with the tumor. The tumor is then resected from the posterior fossa and the inferomedial, and a large part of the inferolateral triangle, are exposed. Whenever the tumor extends further down and medially onto the clivus, the PCP anteriorly and the apex of the petrous bone posteriorly should be drilled off. The PCP can be drilled off by approaching through the space between the intradural ICA and the IIIrd nerve, while the apex of the petrous bone can be drilled off by approaching through the posteromedial triangle. Following removal of the PCP and the apex of the petrous bone, the petroclinoid ligament can be removed, the tumor totally excised and the VIth nerve visualized in its central segment in the posterior fossa and in Dorello's canal. It is evident that the position of the patient's head during drilling of the PCP is anteroposterior, while during drilling of the apex of the petrous bone it is lateral. For this reason, the operating table should be movable in all directions. The intradural portion of the tumor can only be resected when it is possible to follow the ICA from the dural ring around the anterior loop toward the proximal ring and then along the horizontal segment on the medial aspect of the ICA toward the medial loop of the ICA. After identification of the MHT, dissection of the ICA along its segment from the medial loop toward the lateral loop is very difficult unless the VIth nerve has been identified. When the nerve is identified, it is advisable to follow it along the lateral aspect of the horizontal segment of the ICA in Parkinson's triangle toward the SOF compartments where it is on the under aspect of V1. Once the VIth nerve is dissected in addition to the ICA, complete excision of the tumor can be easily accomplished. If the VIth nerve or the IVth nerve were destroyed by the tumor or accidentally injured at surgery, either of them can be reconstructed directly or by using grafts and sutures, or fibrin glue.

In cases of intracavernous tumors and particularly in soft tissue tumors such as pituitary tumors extending into the CS. craniopharyngiomas and chordomas, it is better to use different approaches through different triangles and combinations of them rather than opening the whole CS by excising the entire lateral wall. This is of course not possible in very fibrous and hard meningiomas or in cases of trigeminal neurinomas in which the whole lateral wall of the CS should be excised and the tumor removed from the CS.

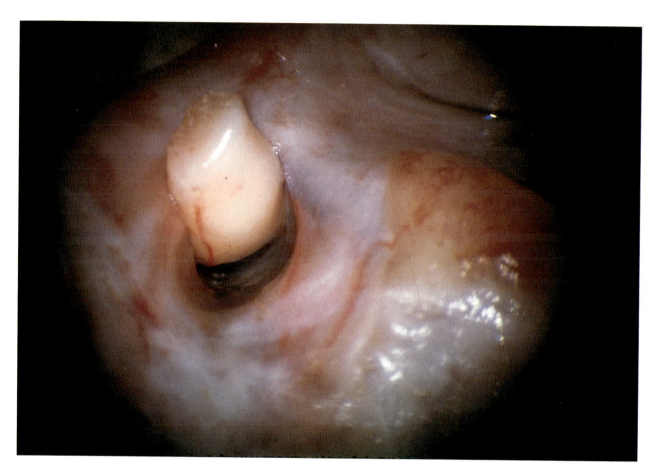

Fig. 142. On a fresh cadaver specimen with injection into the arterial and venous system, the entry point of the IIIrd nerve on the left side is shown under the microscope. The entrance to the nerve canal is located on the lateral aspect of the PCP. It is evident that the entrance into the canal is much larger than the nerve if compared in cross sections. The spare space at the entry point around the nerve facilitates the ingrowth of a meningioma into the canal around the nerve

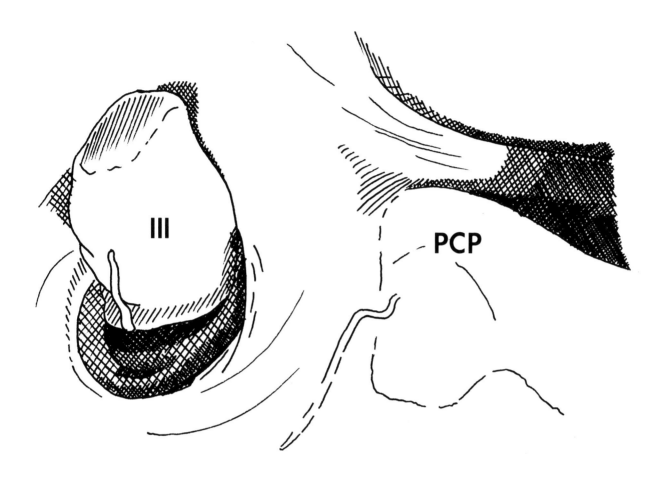

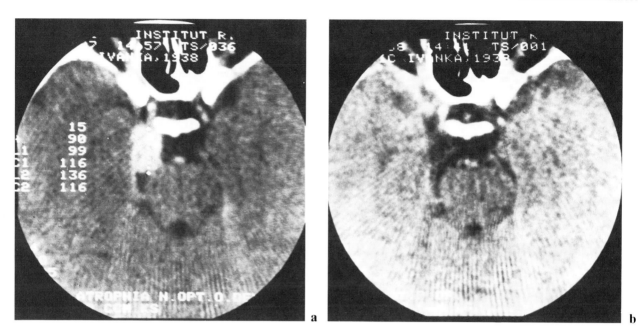

Fig. 143. Axial CT scan of a small meningioma located on the medial aspect of the CS on the left side extending from the entry point of the IVth nerve to the entry point of the IIIrd nerve. The meningioma has grown into the canal of the IIIrd nerve. **a** Preoperative, **b** postoperative

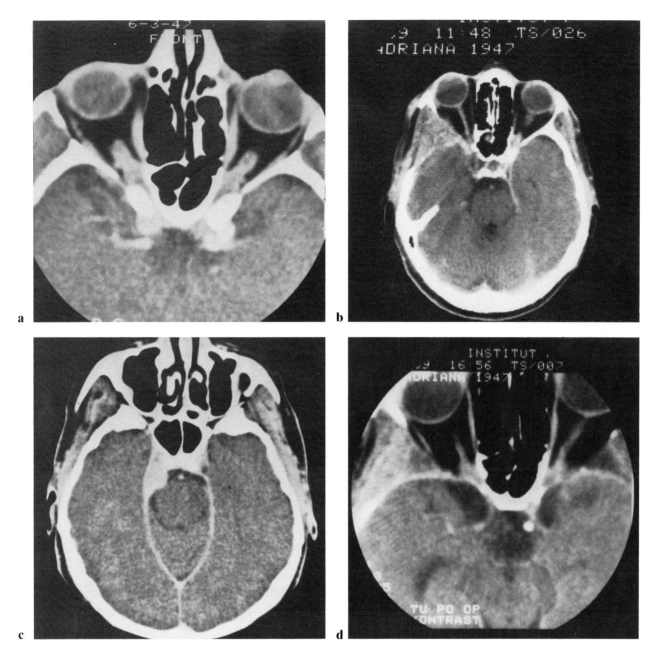

Fig. 144. Contrast-enhanced axial CT scan, preoperative (**a, c**), postoperative (**b, d**). The tumor is located in both orbits, in both optic canals, on the diaphragm of the sella, around both ACPs, and in the left CS (**a, c**). The patient was operated on in two stages. In the initial surgery, the tumor was removed from the left CS, the area around the left ACP, the left optic canal and from the left orbit. Three weeks later, the tumor was also removed from the right side. **b** Postoperative CT scan after the initial surgery on the left side demonstrates no tumor in the left CS, around the left ACP, in the left optic canal nor on the diaphragm of the sella whereas the tumor on the right side is still present. **d** CT scan after the second surgery demonstrates no tumor on either side

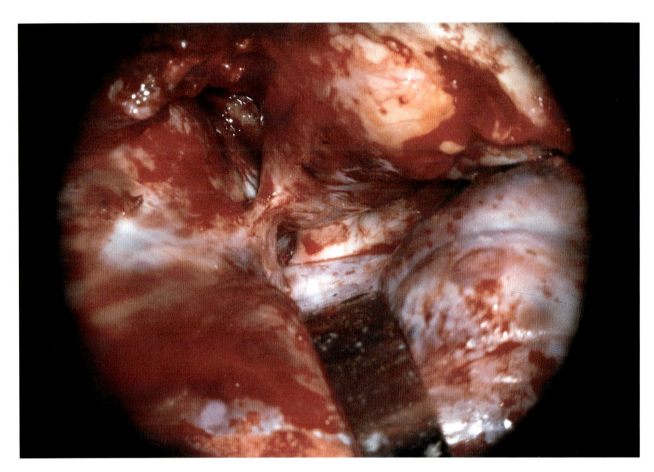

Fig. 145. Intraoperative view during surgery on the left side of the patient presented in Fig. 144. The orbit has been unroofed, the sphenoid wing with the ACP has been removed. The optic canal has been opened and the ON covered with dura propria has been exposed in the whole length from the dura to the orbit. The dura which covers the frontal and temporal lobes has been exposed. The epidural stage of the operation has been fully completed

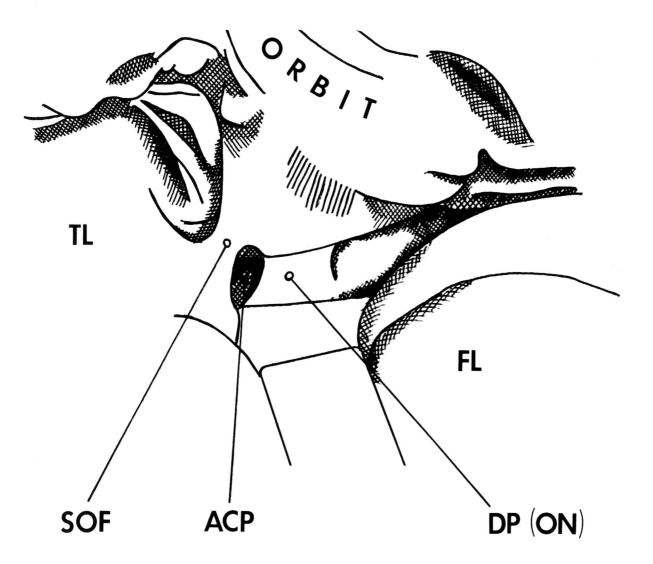

SOF   ACP   DP (ON)

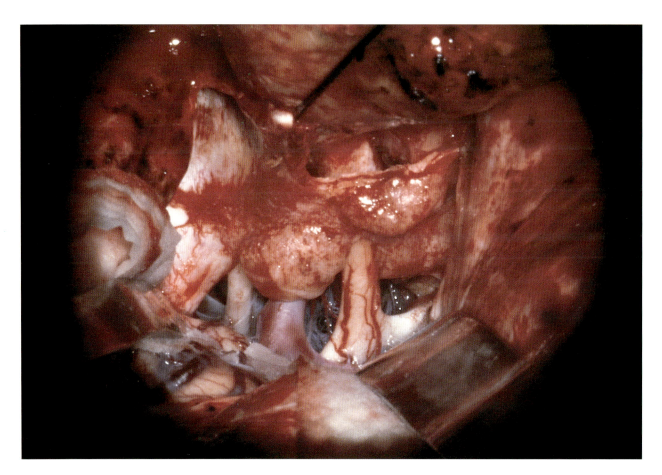

Fig. 146. The dura has been opened along the Sylvian fissure and on the medial aspect of the SOF down to the base of the ACP and then perpendicularly over the ON towards the tuberculum sellae. Intradurally, the left ON with the chiasm, the ICA, the IIIrd nerve, and the lateral wall of the CS are shown. The tumor is attached to the inner aspect of the dura around the ON, the ICA, and the IIIrd nerve, spreading over the lateral wall of the CS

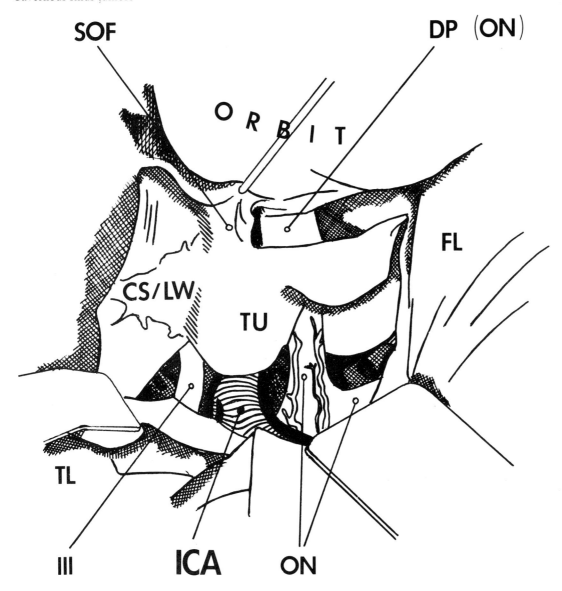

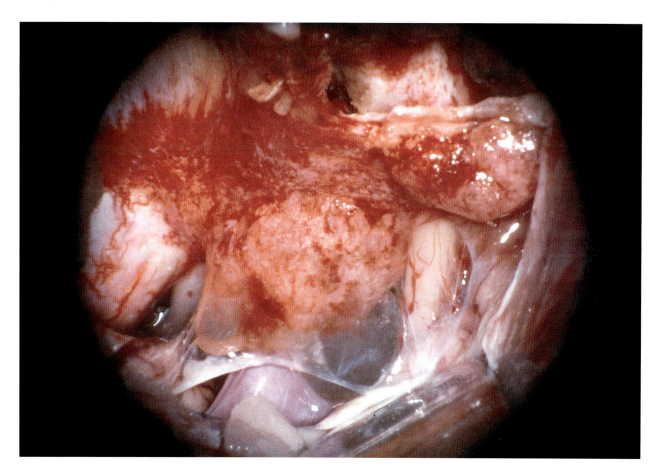

Fig. 147. Under higher magnification the relationships of the tumor, the arachnoidea and structures running through the tumor are shown: the ON, the ICA, and the IIIrd nerve. Note: The anterior part of the lateral wall of the CS is covered by the tumor. Behind the coronal plane at the entry point of the IIIrd nerve, the surface of the lateral wall of the CS is normal

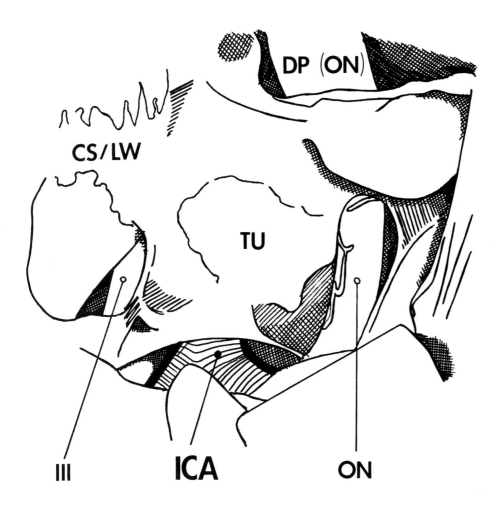

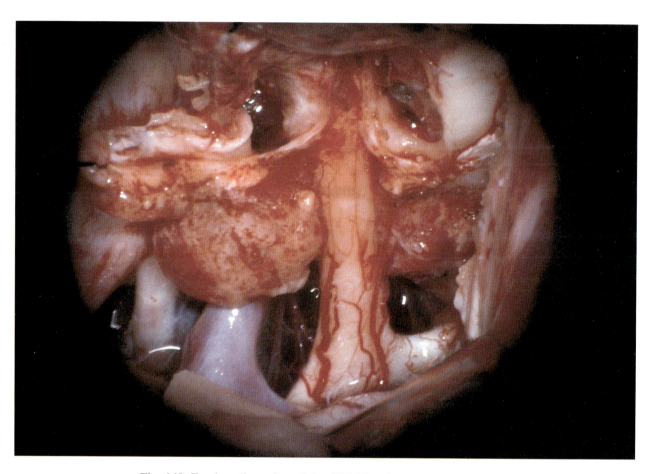

Fig. 148. Further dissection of the ON. The dura propria over the ON in the optic canal is cut along the longitudinal axis of the nerve. The tumor extends along the ON, completely surrounding it throughout the optic canal, and compressing the nerve. Note: The arteries on the ON along its longitudinal axis are preserved

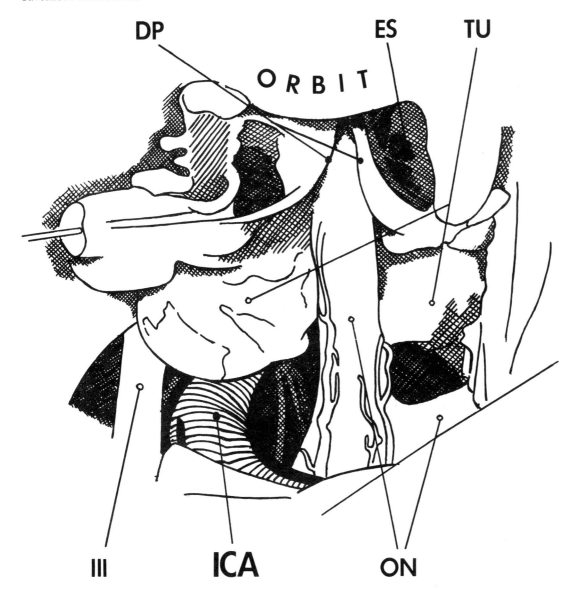

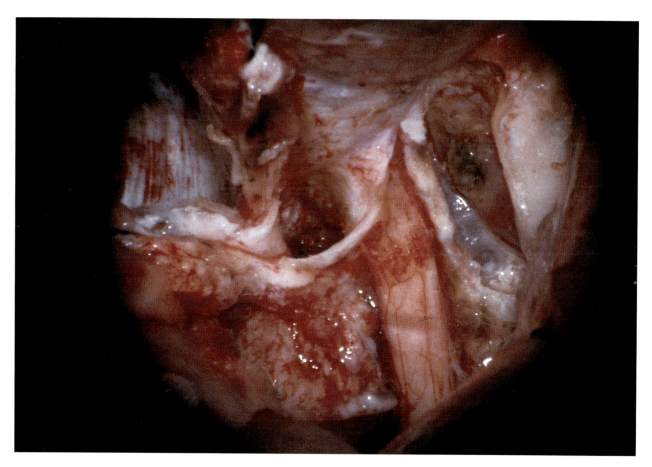

Fig. 149. Longitudinal incision of the dura propria along the longitudinal axis of the ON has been continued to the annulus of Zinn. The tumor around the ON is firmly adherent to the dura propria and the ON. Due to massive expansion of the tumor on the medial aspect of the ON in the optic canal and infiltration of the tumor into the dura propria on the same side, further removal of the wall of the optic canal on the medial aspect has been performed, thus opening the ethmoid cells and exposing the mucous membrane

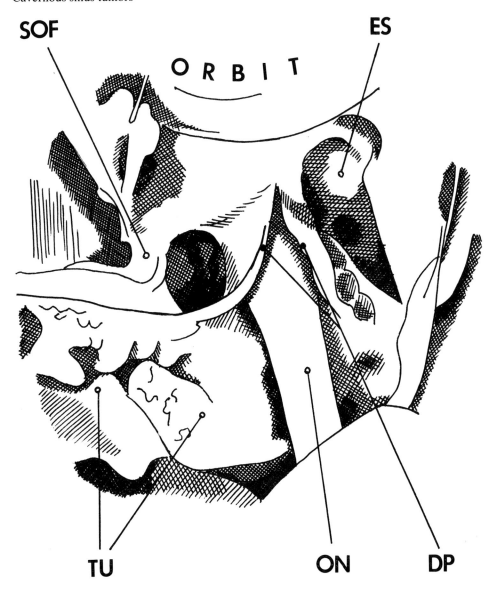

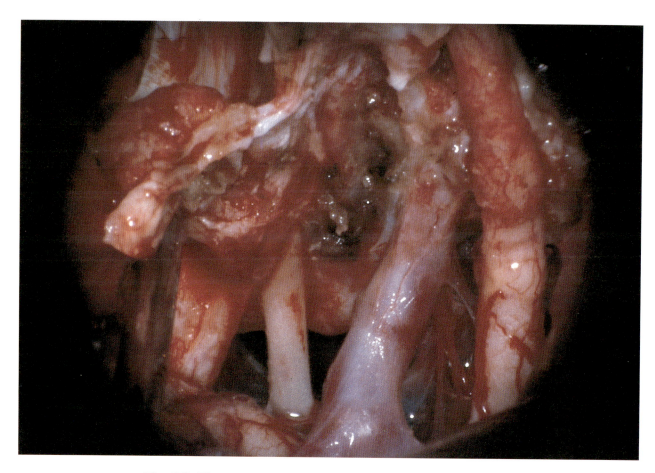

Fig. 150. The tumor has been removed from the ON in the optic canal. The dural ring around the ICA has been excised together with the tumor. The tumor has been removed from the PCP between the ICA and the IIIrd nerve. The anterior loop of the ICA has been exposed. The bulk of the tumor is still in situ, attached to the IIIrd nerve, to the tentorial edge and to the surface of the lateral wall of the CS

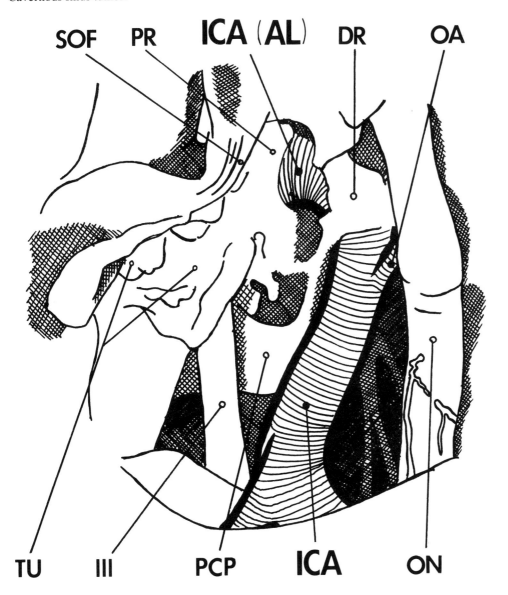

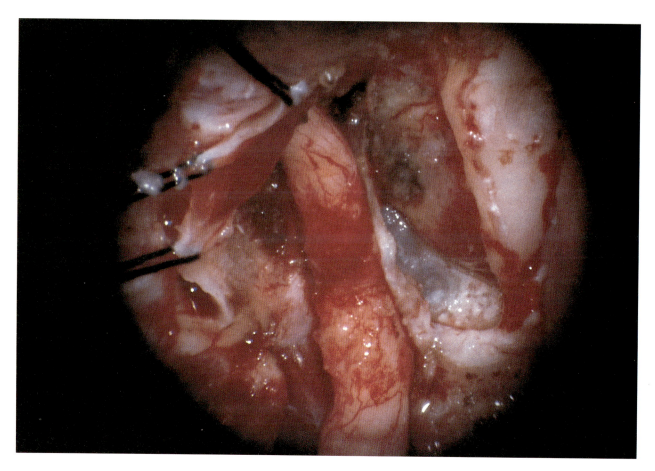

Fig. 151. The ON has been dissected throughout the optic canal, through the annulus of Zinn far into the orbit. The surface of the ON in the optic canal and in the area of the annulus of Zinn is of a non uniform appearance, though the arterial supply to the nerve is preserved. The dura propria, which was invaded by the tumor, has been resected extensively along the ON. On the medial aspect of the nerve, the mucous membrane of the dorsal and lateral cells of the ethmoid sinus is shown. Removal of the tumor around the ON intradurally along the optic canal and in the orbit has been completed

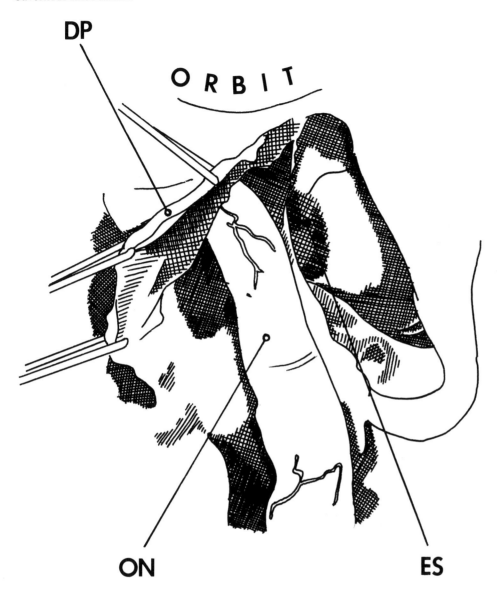

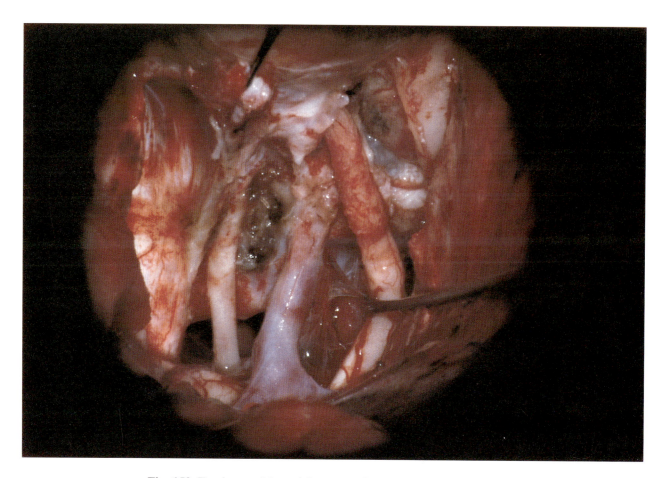

Fig. 152. Further excision of the tumor from the lateral wall of the CS, the SOF structures, the IIIrd nerve intradurally, the anterior loop of the ICA, the area around the PCP, and from the intradural ICA, has been completed. The ON, the ICA, and the IIIrd nerve, i.e., the anteromedial triangle is completely tumor-free

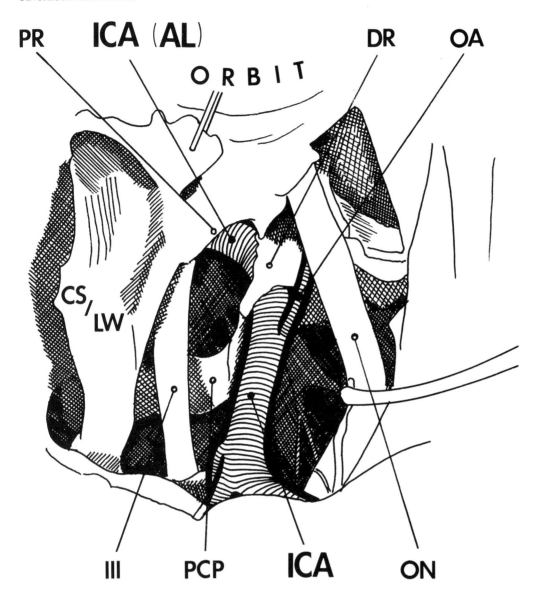

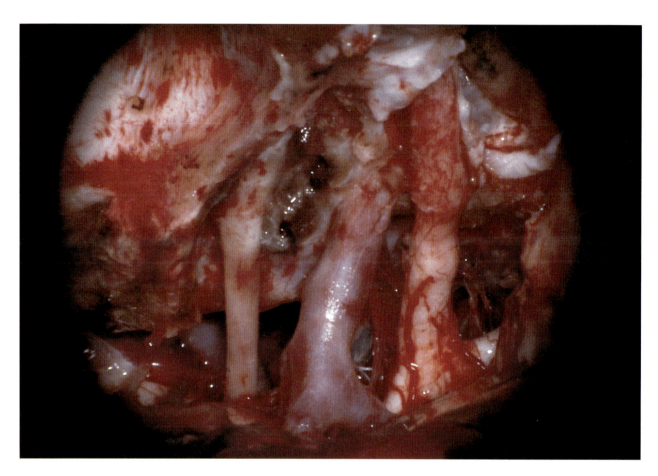

Fig. 153. Further resection of the tumor in the area of the paramedial and Parkinson's triangles has been completed. The tumor has also been removed from the CS. The IIIrd and IVth nerves have been visualized and preserved both in their intradural course and in the lateral wall of the CS towards the orbit. The tumor has been completely removed from the left CS, the left PCP and ACP area, and around the ICA and ON intradurally, around the anterior loop of the ICA in the anteromedial triangle and along the ON throughout the optic canal and in the orbit. Resection of the tumor on the left side is complete and no additional treatment is necessary

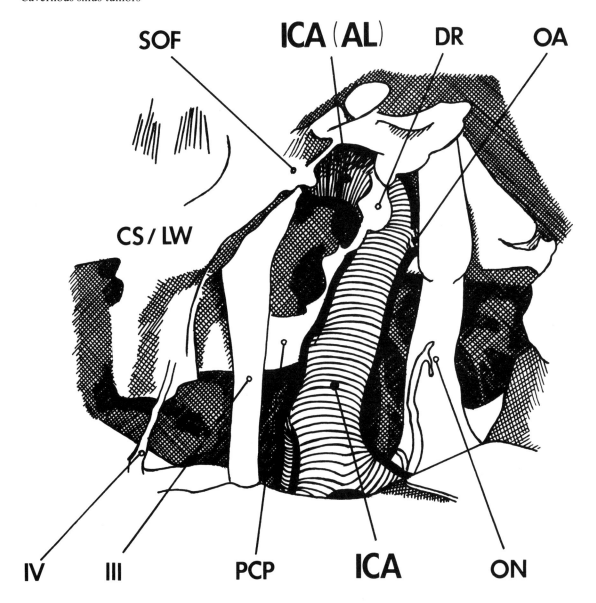

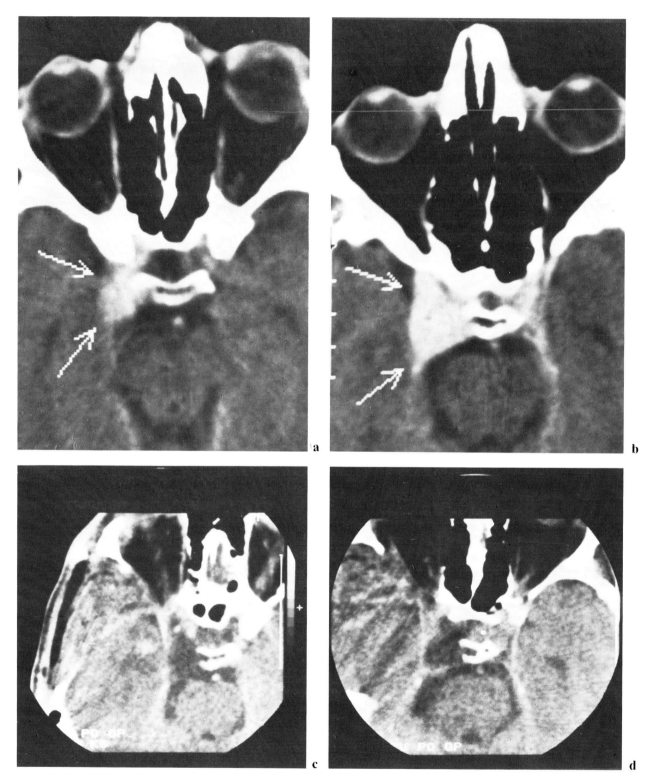

Fig. 154. Contrast-enhanced axial CT scan demonstrating a meningioma on the medial aspect and within the CS on the left side preoperatively (**a, b**), with no residual tumor in the left CS postoperatively (**c, d**)

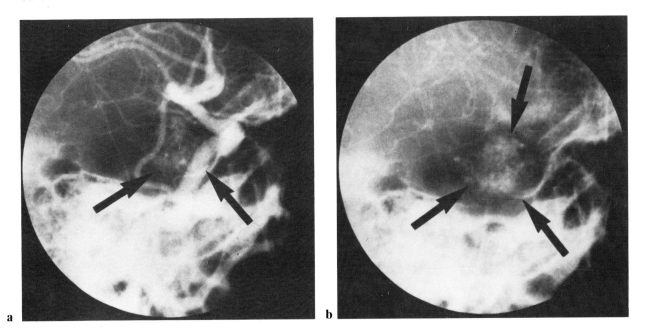

Fig. 155 Left carotid angiograms of the same patient as in Fig. 154, **a, b** demonstrating a rich blood supply to the tumor in the CS, lateral view (**a, b**)

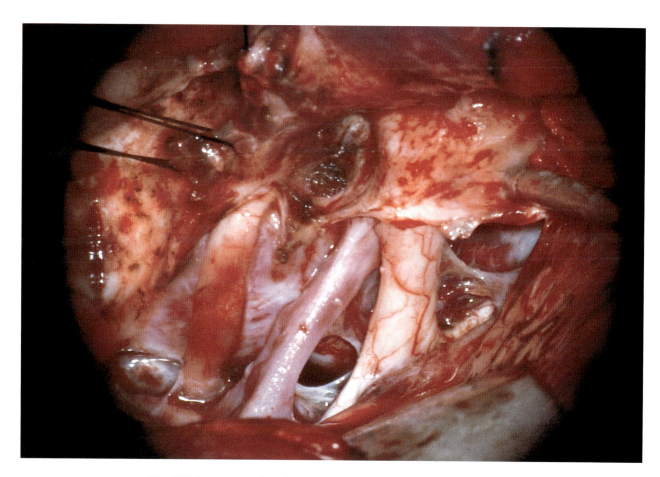

Fig. 156. Intraoperative view of the same patient as in Figs. 154 and 155. The epidural stage of the operation has been completed, the dura being opened in the described way for the approach to the CS and the IIIrd nerve. The ICA and the ON are shown intradurally. The tumor is visualized beneath these three structures on the medial aspect of the CS, still covered by the dura. The ON in the whole segment of the optic canal is visualized and is still covered by the dura propria. The anteromedial triangle has been exposed in its whole extent epidurally. The dura at the base of the triangle has been cut posteriorly over the tumor so that the approach into the CS through the anteromedial triangle is enlarged by incising the dura of the oculomotor trigone

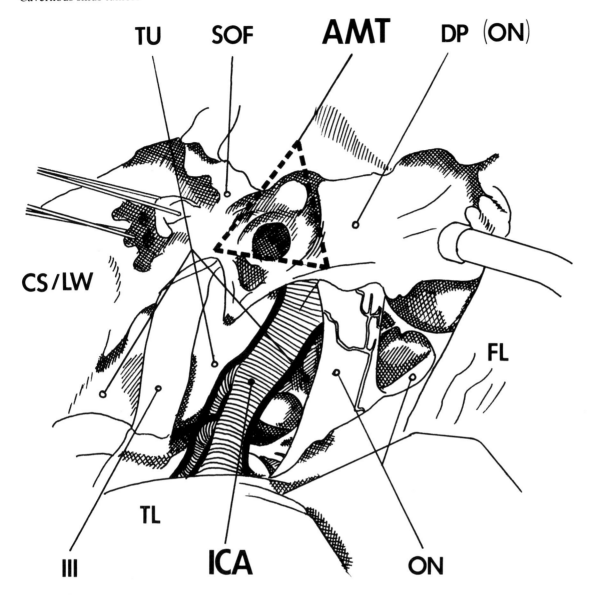

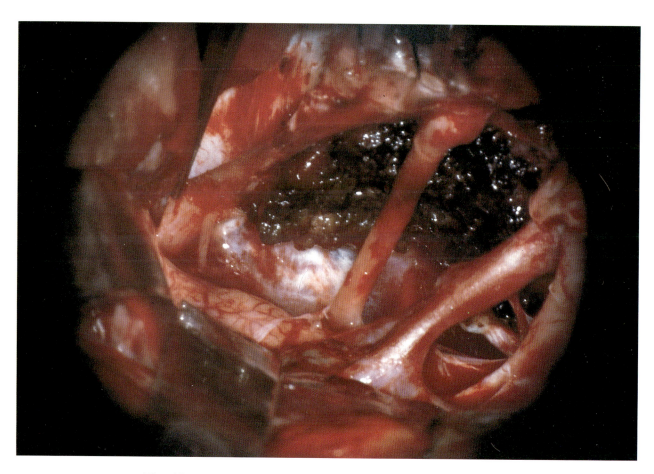

Fig. 157. The tumor has been removed from the CS through the anteromedial and paramedial triangles. Following removal of the tumor, the CS has been packed with Surgicel. The lateral wall of the CS, the IVth and IIIrd nerves, the ICA and the ON are seen to be tumor-free

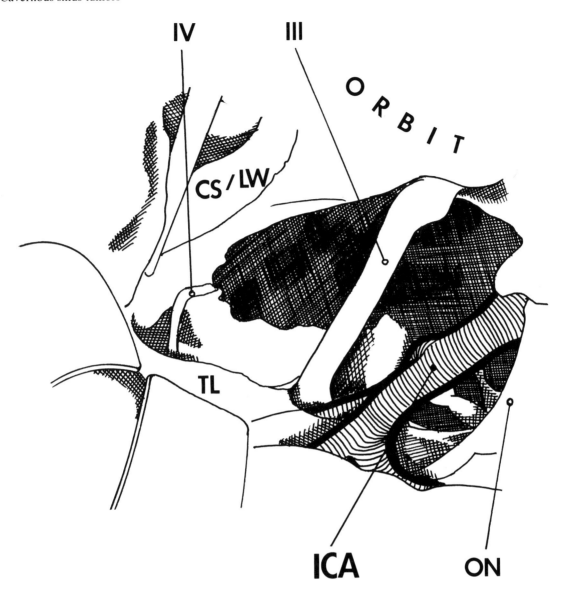

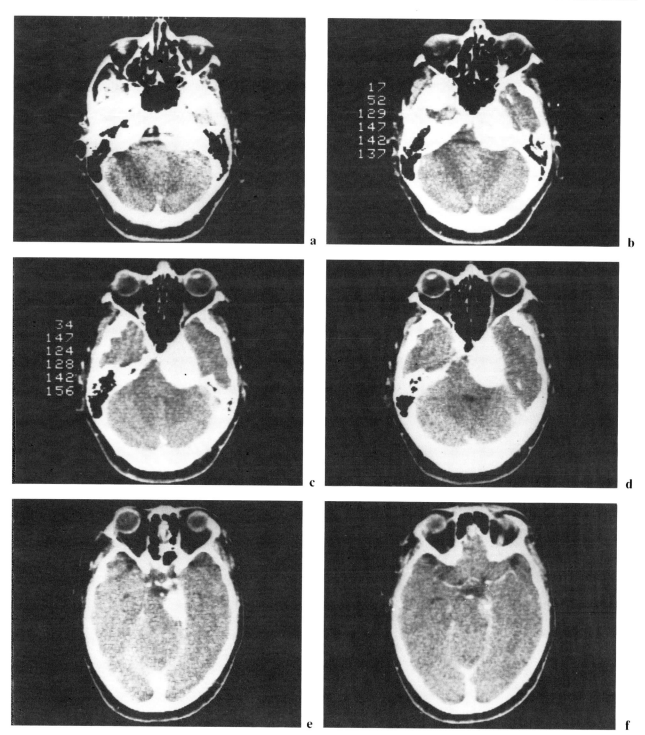

Fig. 158 a–f. Contrast-enhanced serial CT scans demonstrating a large intracavernous tumor on the right side occupying the whole CS and extending into the posterior fossa. A long segment of the brain stem on the right side is compressed by the tumor. The patient was treated by an ophthalmologist for diplopia due to VI nerve paresis five years prior to admission to hospital. Left sided hemiparesis was found due to compression of the brain stem on the contralateral side

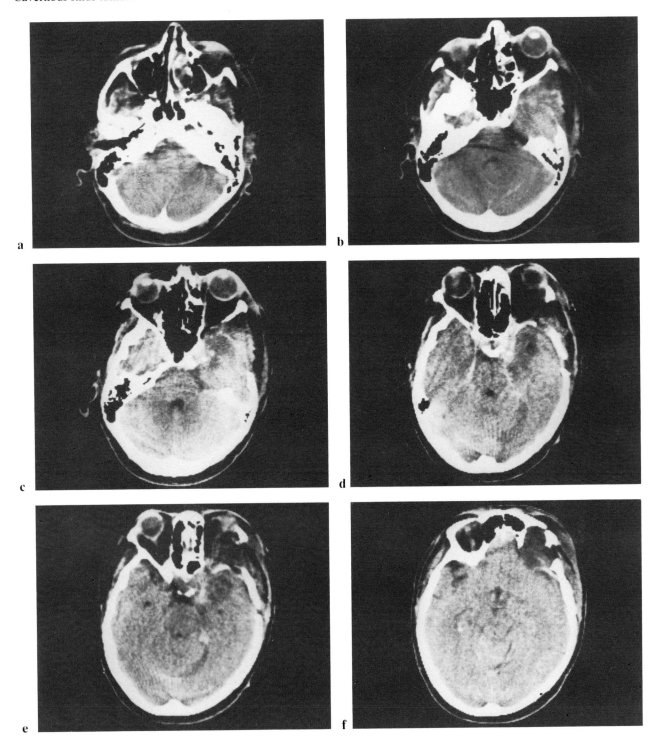

Fig. 159 a–f. Postoperative contrast-enhanced serial CT scans of the same patient as presented in Figs. 158, demonstrating a small residual tumor around the ICA in the right CS

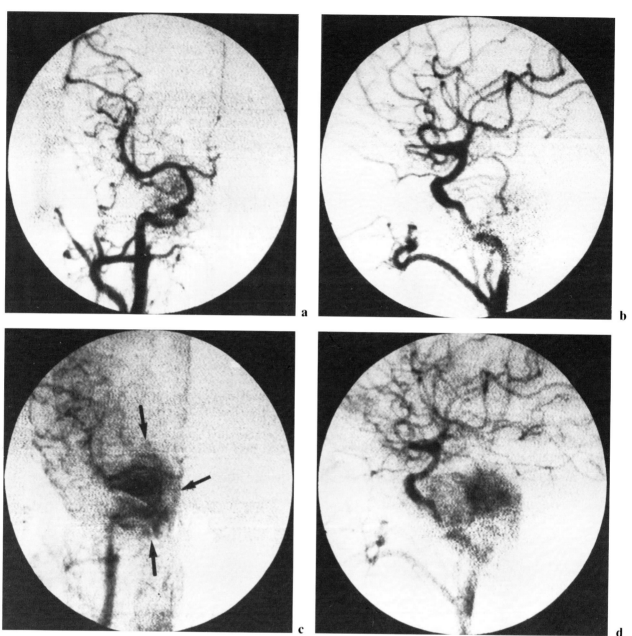

Fig. 160. Preoperative right carotid angiograms AP views (**a, c**) and lateral views (**b, d**) of the same patient as in Figs. 158 and 159, demonstrating a rich blood supply to the tumor in and around the CS. Note:There is no cross flow through the ACoA during compression of the common carotid artery on the left side at the neck (**a**) and there is narrowing of the ICA in the CS in the segment between the lateral and medial loops, indicating invasion of the artery wall by the tumor. Due to absent cross flow through the ACoA and stenosis of the ICA on the right side, the tumor around the ICA in the CS has been left in situ. Postoperative irradiation of the residual tumor was incorporated in the management of this large meningioma

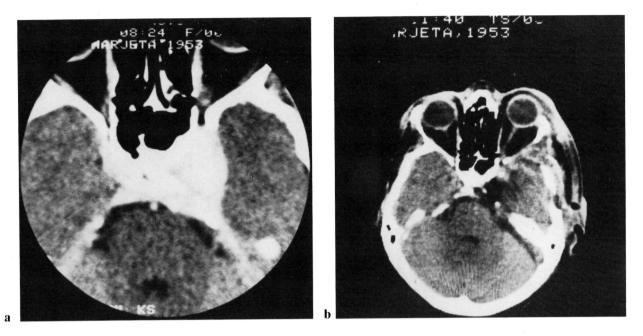

Fig. 161. Contrast-enhanced axial CT scan of an exclusively intracavernous meningioma on the right side, **a** preoperatively, and **b** postoperatively demonstrating no residual tumor

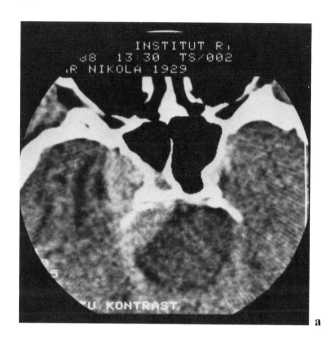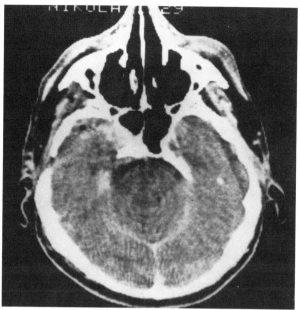

Fig. 162. Contrast-enhanced CT showing a meningioma in the left CS extending into the posterior fossa and compressing the brain stem (**a**), **b** postoperative CT demonstrating no residual tumor

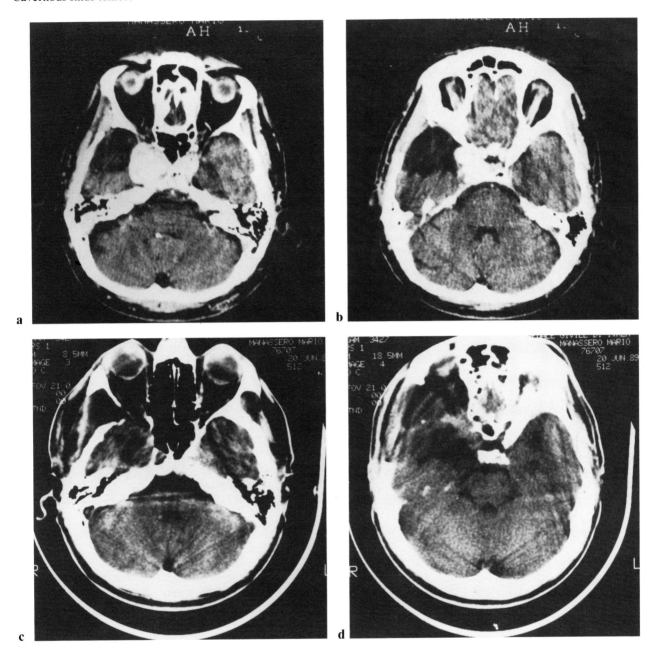

Fig. 163. Contrast-enhanced CT scan demonstrating a meningioma in the right CS (**a, b**) and postoperative CT demonstrating no residual tumor in the right CS (**c, d**). Surgical removal of this tumor is presented step-wise in Figs. 164–171

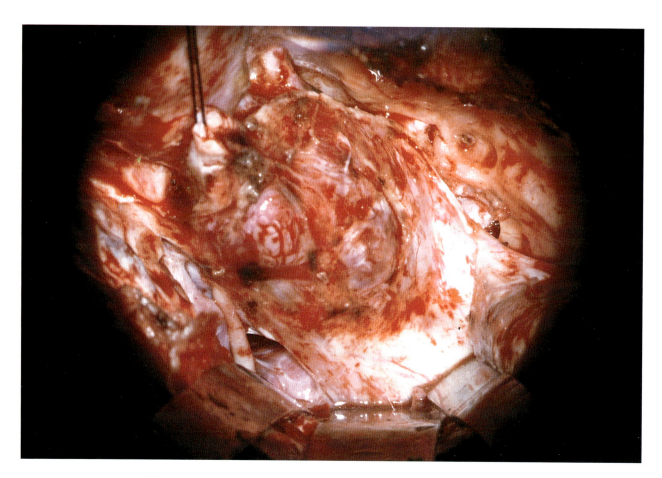

Fig. 164. Following the general approach as described in Chap. 2, the dura has been opened and the temporal lobe retracted. The ON covered with the dura propria in the optic canal, the ON intradurally, the ICA, the PCoA, the IIIrd and the IVth nerves are shown medial to the tentorial edge. The lateral tip of the dura covering the SOF is tied with a suture and fixed anteriorly. V2, V3, the foramen spinosum, with the cut and coagulated proximal stump of the middle meningeal artery, and the ICA in the carotid canal in the petrous bone are shown. The lateral wall of the CS is normal only in the posterior third. The tumor bulges through the anterior two thirds of the lateral wall of the CS

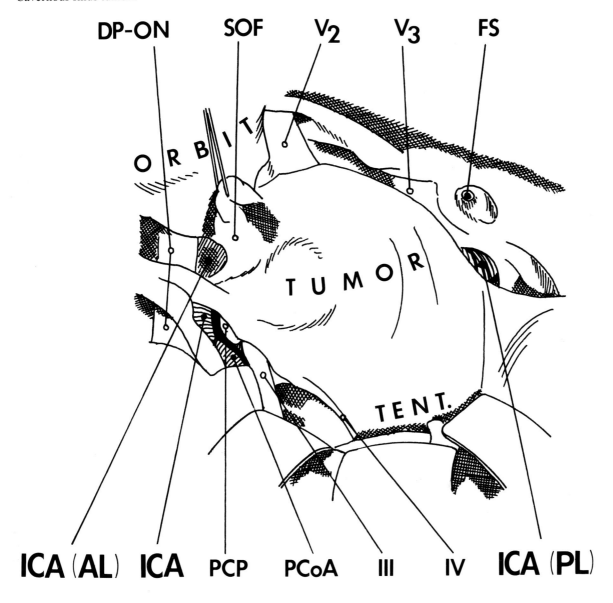

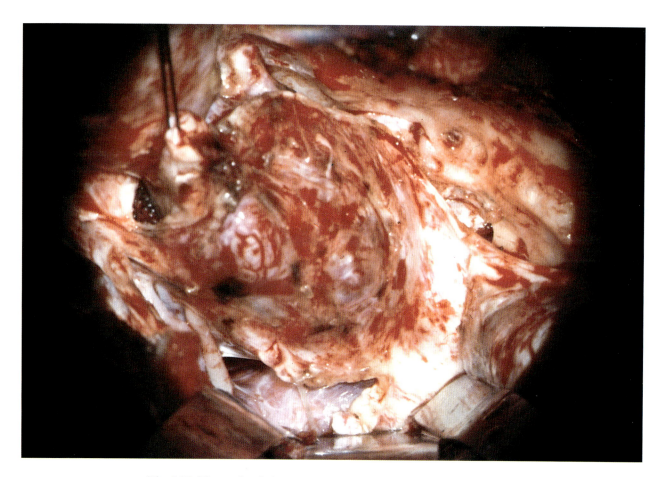

Fig. 165. The patient's head has been placed in the position 3+ (Fig. 67). In such a position, the IVth nerve can be identified and dissected from the edge of the tentorium on its inferior aspect. Following the initial dissection of the IVth nerve, the tentorium has been cut perpendicularly to the IVth nerve in a lateral direction. Such an opening into Parkinson's triangle is very useful to expose the Vth nerve and then to follow it toward the GG, and to ascertain the course of V1, V2, and V3 through the lateral wall of the CS

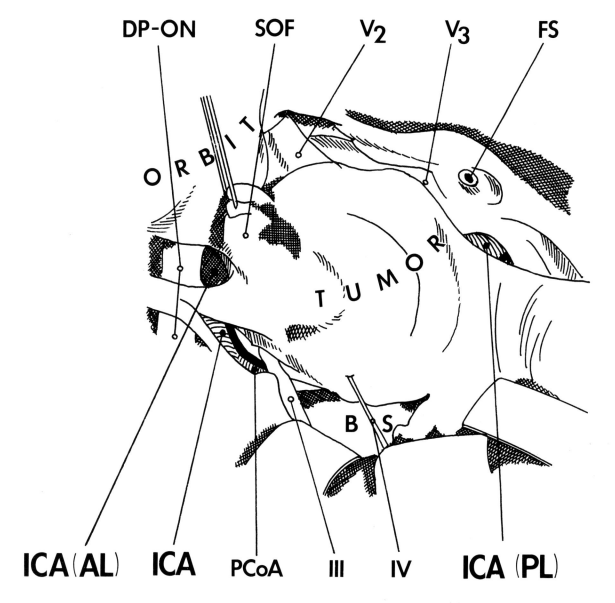

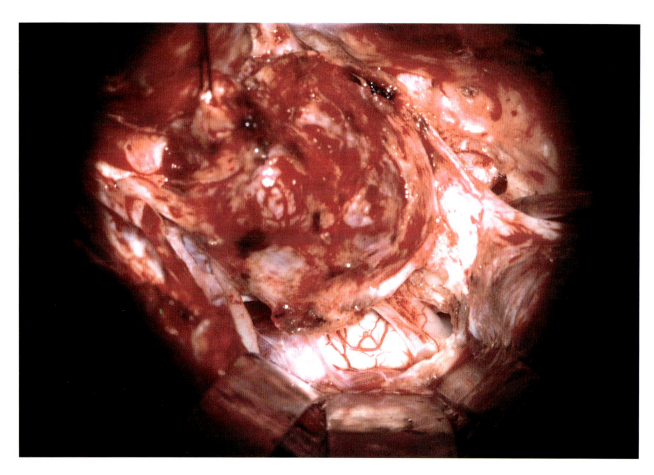

Fig. 166. The outer layer of the CS has been further cut over the Vth nerve and then over the petrous apex and along V3 toward the exit point of V3 from the CS to the foramen ovale. Once the IIIth, IVth, and the Vth nerves have been identified and dissected from the brain stem to the CS, retraction on the temporal lobe can be fully or partially released

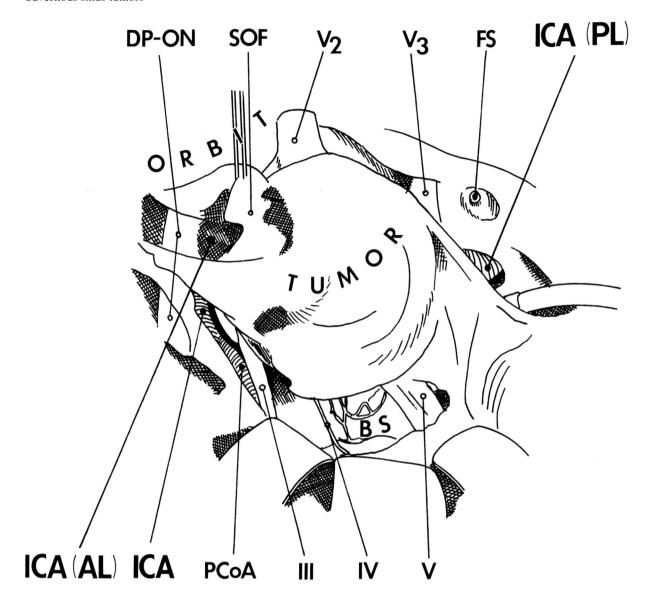

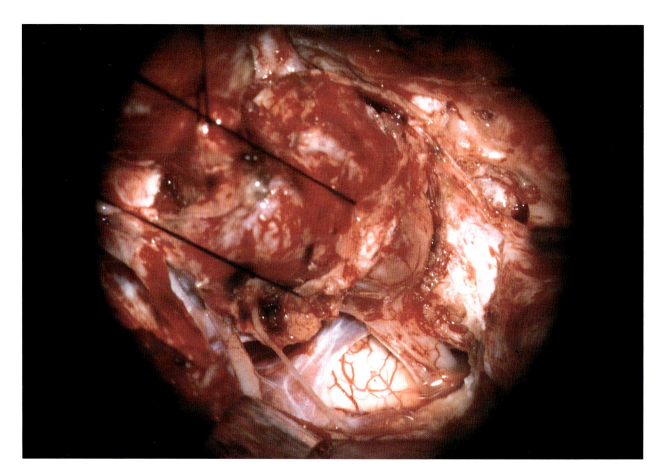

Fig. 167. Further dissection of the IIIth, IVth, and the Vth nerves has been performed. The edges of the outer dural layer of the lateral wall of the CS have been fixed with sutures anteriorly. The outer dural layer has been gently dissected from the trigeminal nerve and the GG. The tumor compresses the GG in a posterior direction towards the apex of the petrous bone and separates V1 from V2. The tumor bulges from the sinus through the apex of the anterolateral triangle

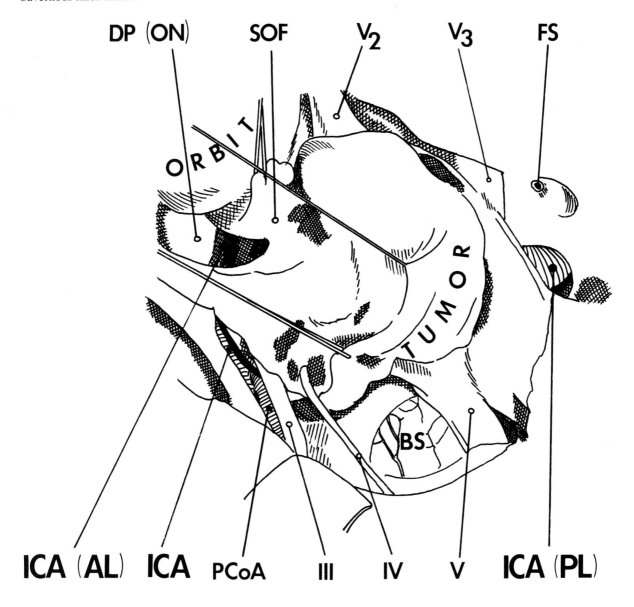

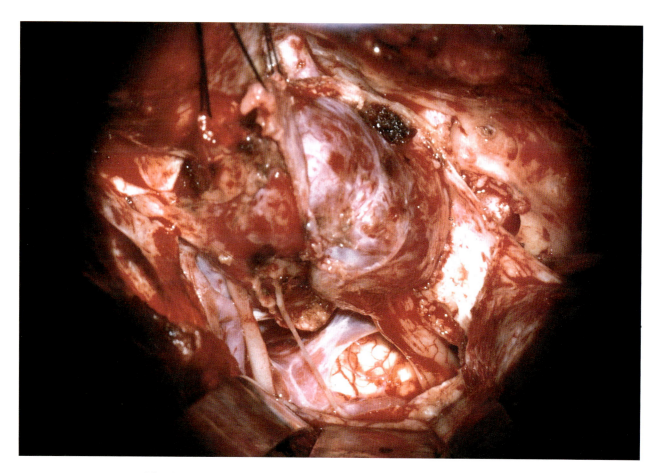

Fig. 168. Further dissection of the IVth nerve has been performed. The outer layer of the lateral wall of the CS has been dissected from the Vth nerve, GG, V1, V2, and V3. The GG, V3, and V2 are pushed in a posterolateral direction while V1 is pushed medially. The tumor bulges through the anterolateral triangle, which is grossly enlarged. Conversely, the lateral triangle is very small. The extensive dissection of the outer layer of the lateral wall from the tumor was easily carried out without any major bleeding

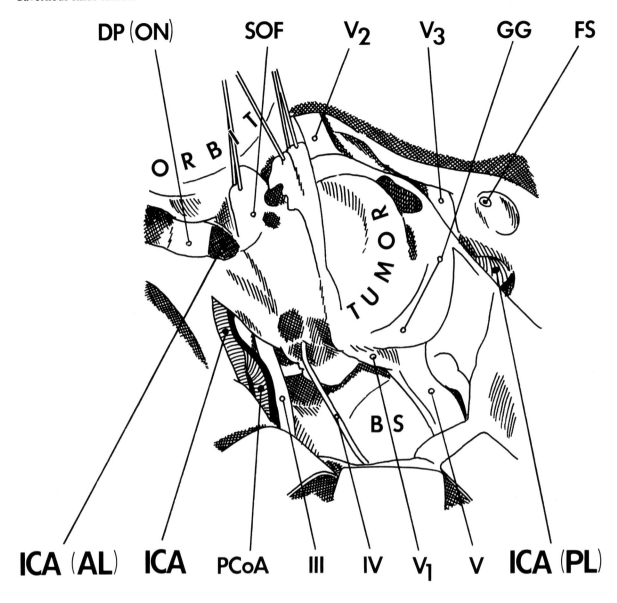

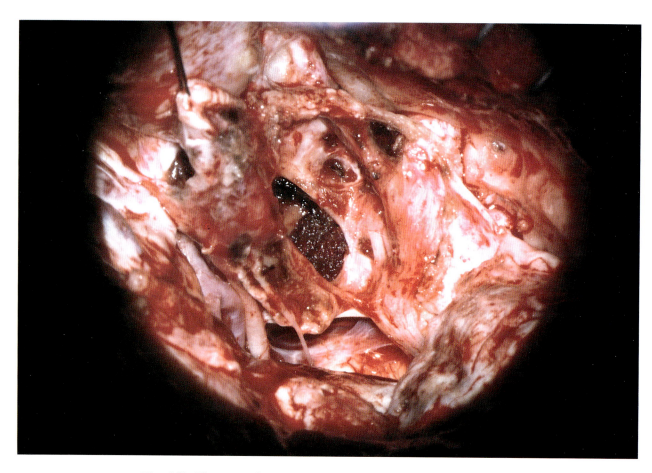

Fig. 169. The tumor has been completely removed from the CS through the anterolateral triangle only. The IIIth, IVth, and the Vth nerves are shown and are tumor-free. The GG is dilated and distorted. V1 is displaced far medially and is atrophic. V3 and V2 are displaced laterally and are also atrophic. The lateral triangle is very small. Through the anterolateral triangle, the lateral ring of the ICA is shown with the ICA underneath, surrounded by Surgicel. The CS is tumor-free

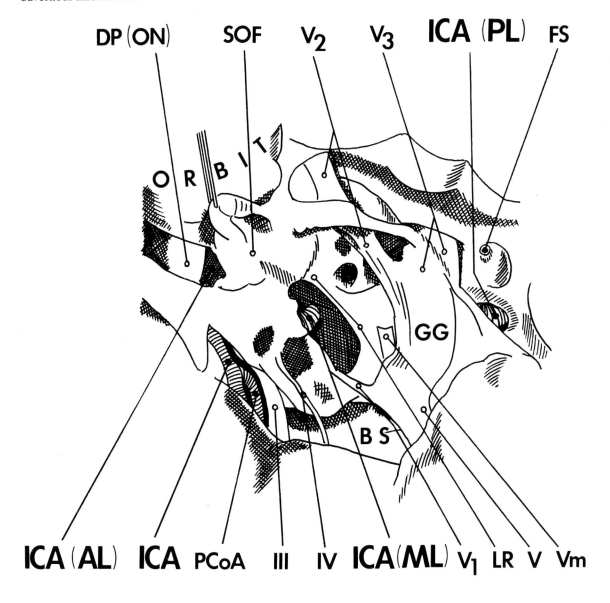

DP (ON) SOF V₂ V₃ ICA (PL) FS

ORBIT

GG

BS

ICA (AL) ICA PCoA III IV ICA (ML) V₁ LR V Vm

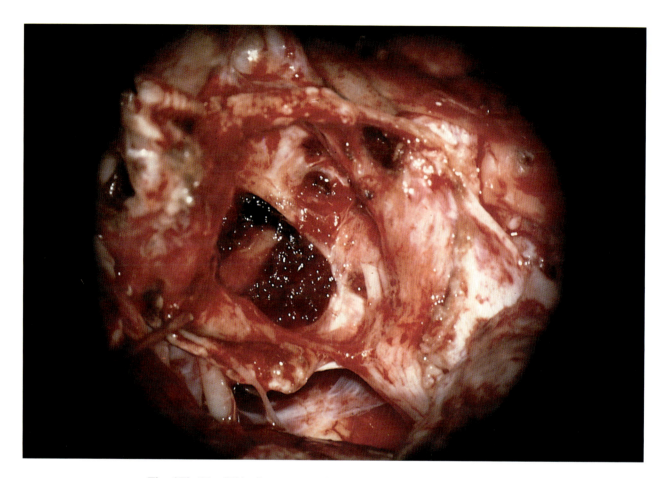

Fig. 170. The CS is shown under higher magnification. The GG is better visualized and it is obviously displaced laterally and flattened. V1 is located far medially. The motor branch of the Vth nerve is seen on the floor of the CS. The lateral ring of the ICA is very large and the space around the ICA under the lateral ring is filled with Surgicel. The ICA is shown in the canal in the petrous bone on the posterior aspect of V3 and in the CS, so one can trace the course of the ICA underneath the GG, running over the foramen lacerum, where it forms the lateral loop

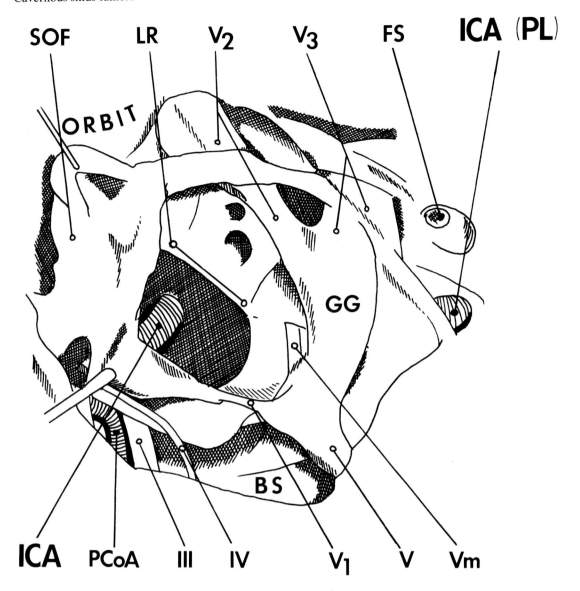

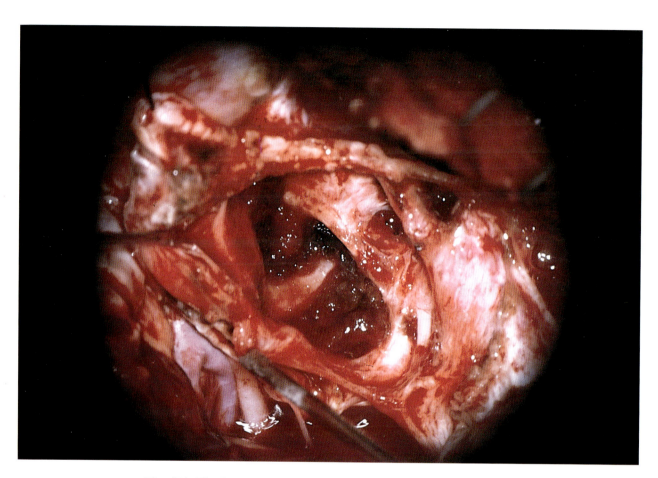

Fig. 171. The interior of the CS has been inspected after complete removal of the tumor and the VIth nerve has been identified on the lateral aspect of the horizontal segment of the ICA running towards the SOF. After dissection of all the structures and complete removal of the tumor, Surgicel has been placed around the ICA and minor venous bleeding arising from the intercavernous sinuses underneath the anterior loop of the ICA has been completely stopped

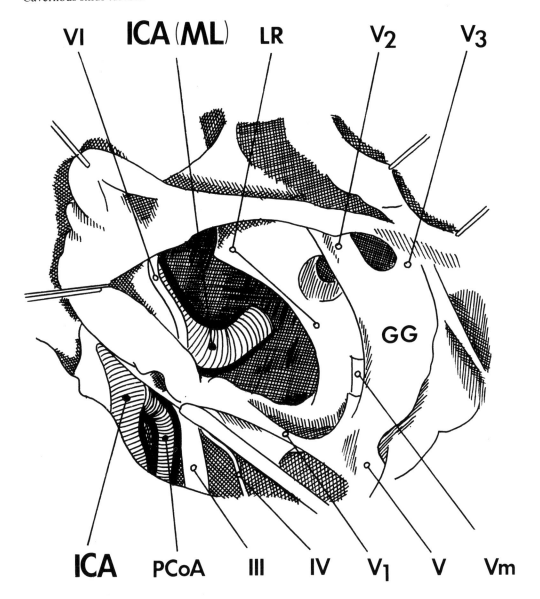

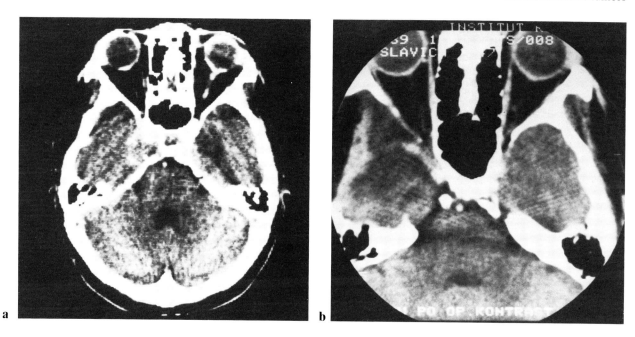

Fig. 172. Contrast-enhanced CT scan demonstrating a tumor in the left parasellar area and in the sella preoperatively (**a**) and no residual tumor postoperatively (**b**). The nature of the tumor was obvious at surgery and the diagnosis of a chordoma confirmed histologically

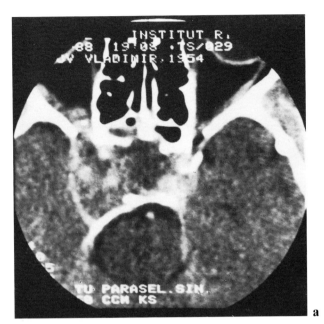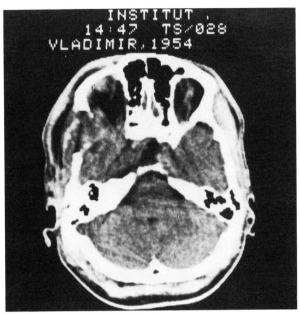

Fig. 173. Contrast-enhanced CT scan showing a left CS tumor preoperatively (**a**) and no residual tumor postoperatively (**b**). The density of the tumor is irregular and not as hyperdense as is usually seen with meningiomas. Surgical excision of the tumor (chordoma) in this patient is presented in Figs. 174–177

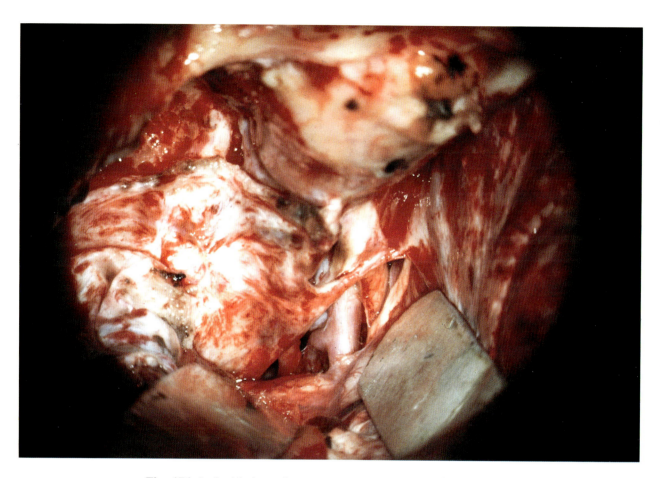

Fig. 174. Left sided craniotomy, characteristic of the approach for intracavernous sinus surgery, has been completed in its epidural stage as described in Chap. 2, and the dura has been opened in the usual way. The lateral wall of the left CS bulges outwards, indicating a tumor in the CS. V2, the unroofed orbit, the dura covering the nerves running from the left CS to the orbit, the anteromedial triangle, and the ON covered with dura propria are shown apidurally. The ON, the ICA with the ACoA, the IIIrd nerve, and the anterior part of the tentorial edge are shown intradurally

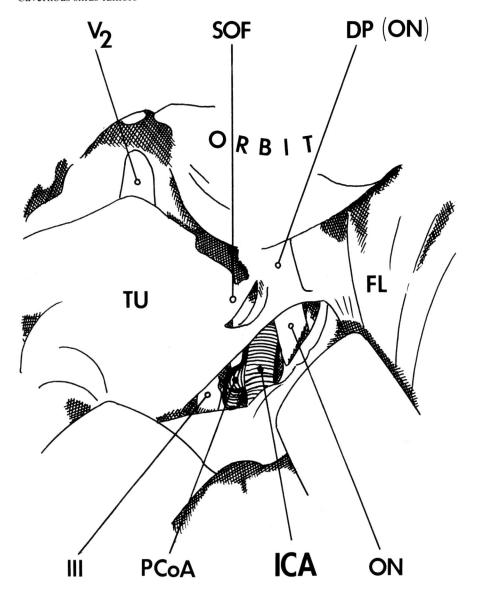

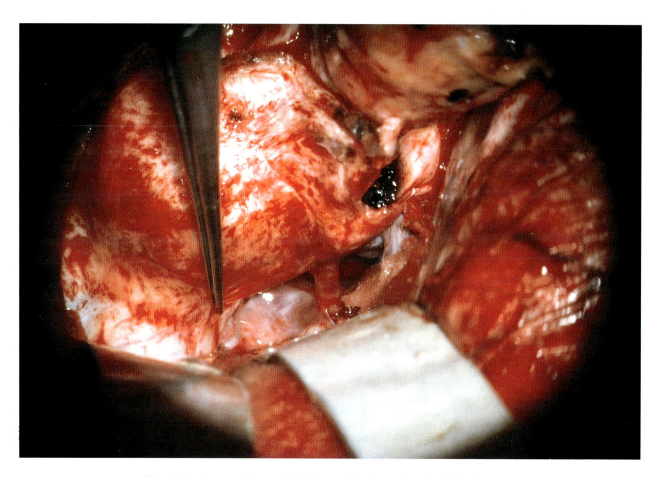

Fig. 175. A round-shaped bulging of the lateral wall of the CS in its anterior two thirds is shown. The posterior third of the left lateral wall of the CS is of normal appearance. The edge of the tentorium has been retracted with microforceps and the IVth nerve is visualized on the inferior aspect of the tentorium. The brain stem, the IIIrd nerve, PCP, and the ICA are seen intradurally. Extradurally, the ON covered with dura propria, the anteromedial triangle and the dura covering the nerves running from the left CS to the orbit, and the orbit itself are shown

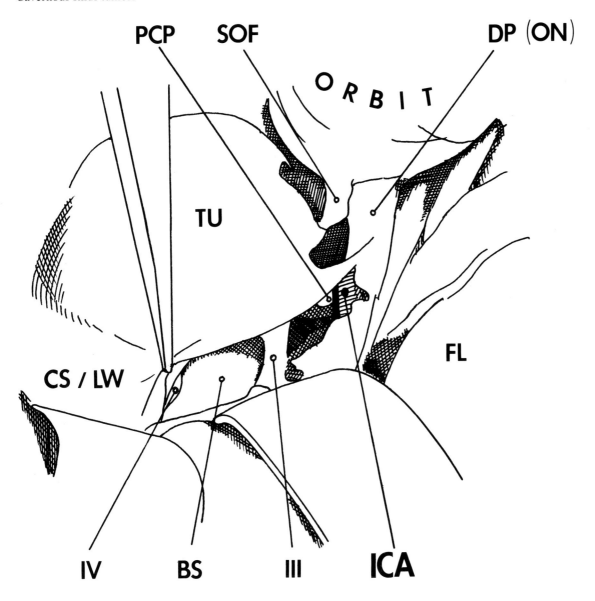

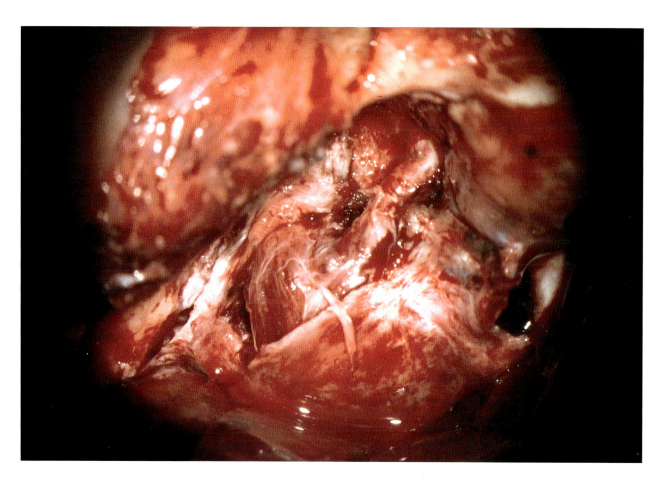

Fig. 176. The head is in the position 2+ (Fig. 67). V2 and V3 have been dissected from the foramen rotundum and foramen ovale, respectively, to the GG. The outer layer of the lateral wall of the CS has been partially removed. V2, V3 and the GG are stretched over the tumor. The tumor is shown in the anterolateral and lateral triangles

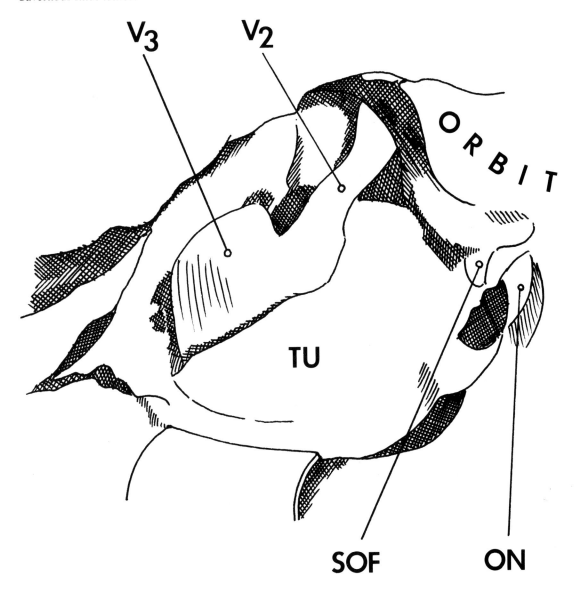

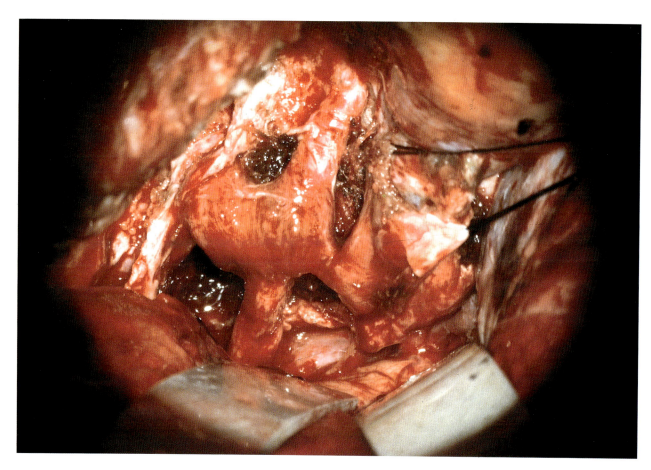

Fig. 177. The left CS has been entered through all the triangles, and the tumor completely removed. The ICA is shown in the anterolateral triangle. Surgicel has been placed around the ICA throughout its entire course through the CS underneath the nerves. The Vth nerve with its branches V1, V2, and V3 and the GG are shown tumor-free

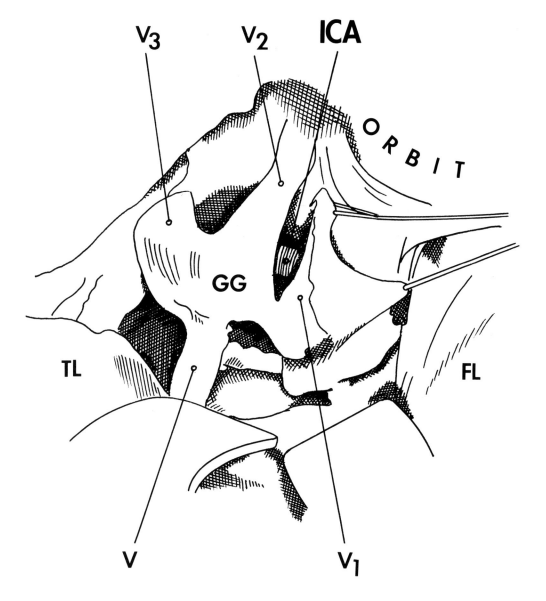

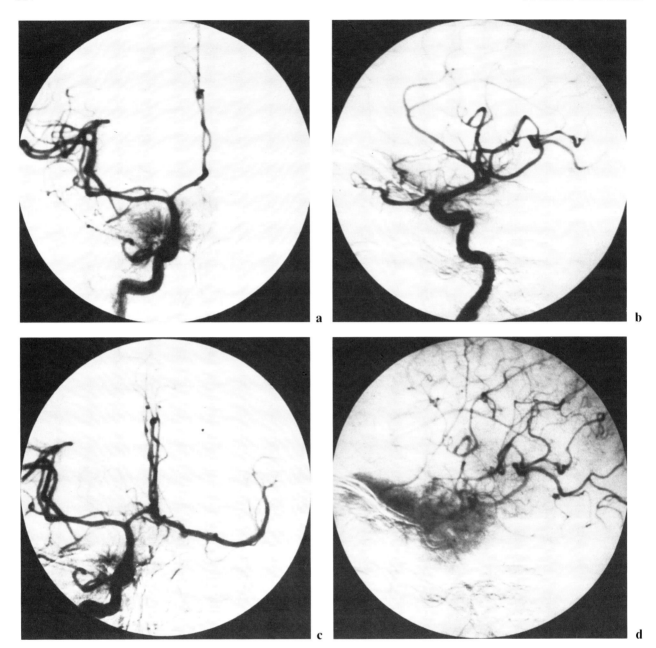

Fig. 178. Right-carotid angiography AP view (**a, c**) and lateral view (**b, d**) demonstrating a characteristic flush of a meningioma in the CS. Cross flow study shows good filling of the left carotid arterial tree from the right side, indicating functional patency of the ACoA (**c**). Extensive arterial flush indicates extension of the tumor in all directions (**d**)

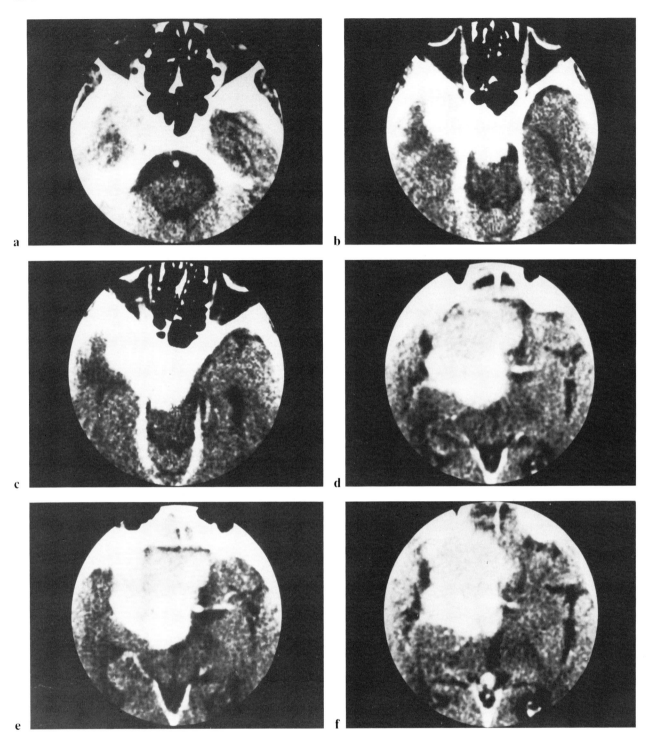

Fig. 179 a–f. Contrast-enhanced serial preoperative CT scans of the same patient as presented in Fig. 178 show a large tumor in the left middle cranial fossa extending throughout the CS into the sella, into the posterior fossa where it compresses the brain stem, and into the anterior fossa and into the brain substance. The tumor, though histologically a benign meningioma, behaves in a malignant fashion. The invasion of the CS in this case was through the whole area of the lateral wall of the CS

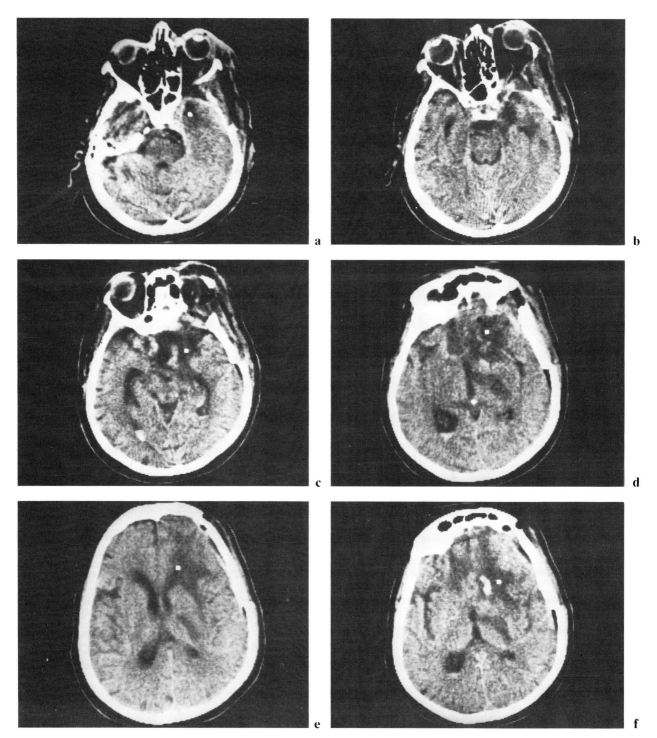

Fig. 180 a–f. Contrast-enhanced serial postoperative CT scans of the same patient as in Figs. 178 and 179, demonstrating a small residual tumor in the CS around the ICA, while the main portion of the tumor has been completely removed

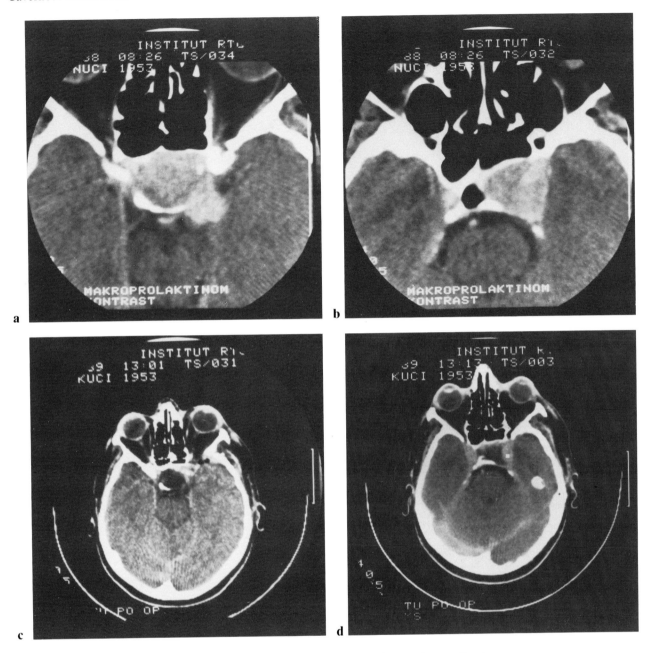

Fig. 181. Contrast-enhanced preoperative CT scans demonstrating an intrasellar tumor with extension into the right parasellar region (**a, b**) and postoperative CT scans (**c, d**) demonstrating no residual tumor, and normal CSs on both sides. This patient was treated with bromocryptine preoperatively with no effect, necessitating surgery

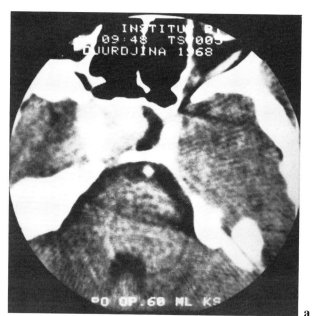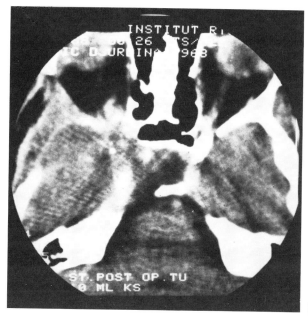

Fig. 182. Contrast-enhanced CT scans demonstrating a left parasellar and partially intrasellar tumor preoperatively (**a**) and no residual tumor postoperatively (**b**). This patient had been operated on two years previously. The initial operation was performed using a transsphenoidal approach to the sella. At the initial surgery part of the tumor was left in the left CS. This later grew and caused symptoms due to compression of the nerves III through VI on the left side. The histological diagnosis of a pituitary adenoma was identical at both operations

References

1. Araki C, Handa S, Handa J, Yoshida K (1965) Traumatic aneurysm of the intracranial portion of the internal carotid artery. J Neurosurg 23: 64–67
2. Benoit BG, Wortzman G (1973) Traumatic cerebral aneurysms: clinical features and natural history. J Neurol Neurosurg Psychiatry 36: 127–13
3. Brassier G, Lasjaunias P, Geugan Y, Pecker J (1987) Microsurgical anatomy of the intracavernous internal carotid artery. In: Dolenc VV (ed) The cavernous sinus. A multidisciplinary approach to vascular and tumorous lesions. Springer, Wien New York, pp 81–103
4. Browder J (1937) Treatment of carotid artery-cavernous sinus fistula. Report of a case. Arch Ophthalmol 18: 95–102
5. Dandy WE, Follis RH Jr (1941) On the pathology of carotid-cavernous aneurysms (pulsating exophthalmos). Am J Ophthalmol 24: 365–385
6. Debrun G (1983) Treatment of traumatic carotid-cavernous fistula using detachable balloon catheters. AJNR 4: 355–365
7. Dolenc VV (1983) Direct microsurgical repair of intracavernous vascular lesions. J Neurosurg 58: 824–831
8. Dolenc VV (1985) A combined epi- and subdural direct approach to carotidophthalmic artery aneurysms. J Neurosurg 62: 667–672
9. Dolenc VV, Škrap M, Šušteršič J, Škrbec M, Morina A (1987) A transcavernous-transsellar approach to the basilar tip aneurysms. Br J Neurosurg 1: 251–59
10. Glasscock ME (1969) Exposure of the intra-petrous portion of the carotid artery. In: Hamberger CA et al (eds) Disorders of the skull base region. Proceedings of the Tenth Nobel Symposium, Stockholm, 1968. Almqvist & Wiksell, Stockholm, pp 135–143
11. Hamby WB (1966) Carotid-cavernous fistula. CC Thomas, Springfield, OH, pp 9 f, 13
12. Harris FS, Rhoton AL Jr (1976) Anatomy of the cavernous sinus. A microsurgical study. J Neurosurg 45: 169–180
13. Ho KC, Meyer G, Garancis J (1982) Chemodectoma involving the cavernous sinus and semilunar ganglion. Hum Pathol 10: 942–943
14. Hodes JE, Fletcher WA, Goodman DF, Hoyt WF (1988) Rupture of cavernous carotid artery aneurysm causing subdural hematoma and death. J Neurosurg 69: 617–619
15. Hunt WE (1976), Tolosa-Hunt syndrome: one cause of painful ophthalmoplegia. J Neurosurg 44: 544–549
16. Julien J, Ferrer X, Drouillard J (1984) Cavernous sinus syndrome due to lymphoma. Short report. J Neurol Neurosurg Psychiatry 47: 558–560
17. Kawase T, Toya S, Shiobara R, Kimura C, Nakajima H (1987) Skull base approaches for meningiomas invading the cavernous sinus. In: Dolenc VV (ed) The cavernous sinus. A multidisciplinary approach to vascular and tumorous lesions. Springer, Wien New York, pp 346–354

18. Kawase T, Toya S, Shiobara S, Mine S (1985) Transpetrosal approach for aneurysms of the lower basilar artery. J Neurosurg 63: 857–861
19. King LW, Molitch ME, Gittinger JW Jr (1983) Cavernous sinus syndrome due to prolactinoma: resolution with bromocriptine. Surg Neurol 19: 280–284
20. Kline LB, Galbraith JG (1981) Parasellar epidermoid tumor presenting as painful ophthalmoplegia. Case report. J Neurosurg 54: 113–117
21. Knosp E, Meller G, Perneczky A (1987) The blood supply of the cranial nerves in the lateral wall of the cavernous sinus. In: Dolenc VV (ed) The cavernous sinus. A multidisciplinary approach to vascular and tumorous lesions. Springer, Wien New York, pp 67–80
22. Koh CS, Tan CT, Alhady SF (1983) Cavernous sinus syndrome. A manifestation of non-Hodgkin's lymphoma of the ethmoid sinus. Med J Aust 2: 451–452
23. Lang J. (1987) Middle cranial base anatomy. In: Sekhar LN et al (eds) Tumors of the cranial base. Diagnosis and treatment. Futura, Mount Kisco, NY, pp 313–334
24. Lenzi GL, Fieschi C (1977) Superior orbital fissure syndrome. Review of 130 cases. Eur Neurol 16: 23–30
25. Lesoin F, Pellerin P, Autricque A, Clarisse J, Jomin M (1987) The direct microsurgical approach to intracavernous tumors. In: Dolenc VV (ed) The cavernous sinus. A multidisciplinary approach to vascular and tumorous lesions. Springer, Wien New York, pp 323–331
26. Lie TA (1968) Congential anomalies of the carotid arteries, including the carotid-basilar and carotid-vertebral anastomoses. An angiographic study and a review of the literature. Excerpta Medica, Amsterdam
27. Maurer JJ, Mills M, German WJ (1961) Triad of unilateral blindness, orbital fracture and massive epistaxis after head injury. J Neurosurg 18: 837–840
28. Mills RP, Insalaco SJ, Joseph A (1981) Bilateral cavernous sinus metastasis and ophthalmoplegia. Case report. J Neurosurg 55: 463–466
29. Mullan S (1979) Treatment of carotid-cavernous fistulas by cavernous sinus occlusion. J Neurosurg 50: 131–144
30. Newton TH, Hoyt WF (1970) Dural arteriovenous shunts in the region of the cavernous sinus. Neuroradiology 1: 71–81
31. Obrador S, Gomez-Bueno J, Silvela J (1974) Spontaneous carotid-cavernous fistula produced by ruptured aneurysm of the internal carotid artery. Case report. J Neurosurg 40: 539–543
32. Odom GL (1964) Ophthalmic involvement in neurological vascular lesions. In: Smith JD (ed) Neuro-ophthalmology. CC Thomas, Springfield, OH, pp 1–96
33. Ono M, Ono M, Rhoton AL Jr (1984) Microsurgical anatomy of the region of the tentorial incisure. J Neurosurg 60: 365–399
34. Parkinson D (1964) Collateral circulation of cavernous carotid artery: anatomy. Can J Surg 7: 251–268
35. Parkinson D (1965) A surgical approach to the cavernous portion of the carotid artery. Anatomical studies and case report. J Neurosurg 23: 474–483
36. Parkinson D (1973) Carotid cavernous fistula: direct repair with preservation of the carotid artery. Technical note. J Neurosurg 38: 99–106
37. Parkinson D (1988) Surgical management of internal carotid artery aneurysms within the cavernous sinus. In: Schmidek HH et al (eds) Operative neurosurgical techniques. Indications, methods and results. Grune & Stratton, Orlando, FL, pp 837–844
38. Peeters FLM, Kroeger R (1979) Dural and direct cavernous sinus fistulas. AJR 132: 599–606
39. Pool JL, Potts DG (1965) Aneurysms and arteriovenous anomalies of the brain: diagnosis and treatment. Harper & Row, New York, p 307
40. Raskind R, Johnson N, Hance D (1977) Carotid cavernous fistula in pregnancy. Angiology 28: 671–676

41. Renn WH, Rhoton AL Jr (1975) Microsurgical anatomy of the sellar region. J Neurosurg 43: 288–198

42. Rhoton AL Jr, Hardy DG, Chambers SM (1979) Microsurgical anatomy and dissection of the sphenoid bone, cavernous sinus and sellar region. Surg Neurol 12: 63–104

43. Serbinenko FA (1974) Balloon catheterization and occlusion of major cerebral vessels. J Neurosurg 41: 125–145

44. Slamovits TL, Cahill KW, Sibony PA, Dekker A, Johnson BL (1983) Orbital fine-needle aspiration biopsy in patients with cavernous sinus syndrome. J Neurosurg 59: 1037–1042

45. Slusher MM, Lennington BR, Weaver RG (1979) Ophthalmic findings in dural arteriovenous shunts. Ophthalmology 86: 720–731

46. Taniguchi RM, Goree JA, Odom GL (1971) Spontaneous carotid-cavernous shunts presenting diagnostic problems. J Neurosurg 35: 384–391

47. Taptas JN (1982) The so-called cavernous sinus: a review of the controversy and its implications for neurosurgeons. Neurosurgery 11: 712–717

48. Thomas JE, Yoss RE (1970) The parasellar syndrome: problems in determining etiology. Mayo Clin Proc 45: 617–623

49. Toya S, Shiobara R, Izumi J (1981) Spontaneous carotid-cavernous fistula during pregnancy or in the postpartum stage. Report of two cases. J Neurosurg 54: 252–256

50. Trobe JD, Glaser JS, Post JD (1978) Meningiomas and aneurysms of the cavernous sinus. Neuroophthalmologic features. Arch Ophthalmol 96: 457–467

51. Umansky F, Nathan N (1987) The cavernous sinus. An anatomic study of its lateral wall. In: Dolenc VV (ed) The cavernous sinus. A multidisciplinary approach to vascular and tumorous lesions. Springer, Wien New York, pp 56–66

52. Unsold R, Safran AB, Safran E (1980) Metastatic infiltration of nerves in the cavernous sinus. Arch Neurol 37: 59–61

53. Vinuela F, Fox AJ, Debrun GM (1984) Spontaneous carotid-cavernous fistulas: clinical, radiological, and therapeutic considerations. Experience with 20 cases. J Neurosurg 60: 976–984

54. Walker AE, Allegre GE (1956) Carotid-cavernous fistulas. Surgery 39: 411–422

55. Yasargil MG, Fox JL, Ray MW (1975) The operative approach to aneurysms of the anterior communicating artery. In: Krayenbühl H (ed) Advances and Technical Standards in Neurosurgery. Springer, Wien New York, Vol. 2, pp 113-170

56. Yasargil MG, Gasser JC, Hodosh RM et al (1977) Carotid-ophthalmic aneurysms: direct microsurgical approach. Surg Neurol 8: 155-165

57. Yasargil MG, Antič J, Laciga R et al (1976) Microsurgical pterional approach to aneurysms of the basilar bifurcation. Surg Neurol 6: 83–89

Subject index